P9-DNV-337

Tell Me What to Eat
If I Have
Irritable Bowel Syndrome

Revised Edition

Nutrition You Can Live With

By Elaine Magee, MPH, RD

Contributions by Christine L. Frissora, MD

New Page Books
A Division of The Career Press, Inc.
Pompton Plains, NJ

Copyright © 2009 by Elaine Magee, MPH, RD

All rights reserved under the Pan-American and International Copyright Conventions. This book may not be reproduced, in whole or in part, in any form or by any means electronic or mechanical, including photocopying, recording, or by any information storage and retrieval system now known or hereafter invented, without written permission from the publisher, The Career Press.

TELL ME WHAT TO EAT IF I HAVE IRRITABLE BOWEL SYNDROME
EDITED AND TYPESET BY GINA TALUCCI
Cover design by Lu Rossman/Digi Dog Design NYC
Printed in the U.S.A.

Contributions by Christine L. Frissora, MD

To order this title, please call toll-free 1-800-CAREER-1 (NJ and Canada: 201-848-0310) to order using VISA or MasterCard, or for further information on books from Career Press.

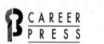

The Career Press, Inc., 220 West Parkway, Unit 12
Pompton Plains, NJ 07444
www.careerpress.com
www.newpagebooks.com

Library of Congress Cataloging-in-Publication Data

Magee, Elaine.
    Tell me what to eat if I have irritable bowel syndrome : nutrition you can live with / by Elaine Magee. —Rev. ed.
        p. cm.
    Includes index.
    ISBN 978-1-60163-020-9
    1. Irritable colon—Popular works. 2. Irritable colon—Diet therapy.
I. Title.
    RC862.I77M24 2009
    616.3′ 42--dc22

                                                                2008022022

Acknowledgments

I am so grateful for the day I found IBS expert Dr. Christine Frissora. Since that day, she has partnered with me for the update on this book, selflessly sharing her knowledge and her enthusiasm every step of the way. It was such a gift to have her input and expertise for the foreword and throughout the rest of the book; she has my deepest thanks and my eternal respect.

Contents

Foreword

A New Look at Irritable Bowel Syndrome (IBS)

Irritable Bowel Syndrome (IBS) is a confusing and mysterious disorder that has many causes and triggers, most of which we don't fully understand. IBS is unpredictable and annoying. The doctors are often as perplexed and frustrated as the patient and the patient's family. This little book offers honest and accurate advice as well as helpful hints about shopping at the grocery store, preparing meals and visiting the doctor's office. I share with you the pearls of wisdom I have gained from treating thousands of patients with IBS for more than a decade. I hope the book, and the resources in it, will help you to live an easier and happier life.

The truth is that IBS has long been misunderstood and misdiagnosed. Although the exact mechanism is not understood, IBS patients suffer from two major problems: increased sensitivity of the gastrointestinal tract and pain and altered movement of the intestine. In IBS the neurons in the intestine are hyper sensitive to "noxious" stimuli [food; gas or distention] and also function in an uncoordinated way resulting in fast and painful activity, slow and bloated activity, or completely unpredictable patterns.

IBS is a disorder in which abdominal pain or discomfort is associated with defecation or a change in bowel habits. Abnormal stool frequency is defined as more than three stools per day or less than three stools per week. IBS patients also report hard or loose watery stool, feelings of incomplete evacuation or retained stool, bloating or abdominal distention, and the passage of mucus.

Approximately 30 percent of patients with IBS have diarrhea as the predominant symptom, 30 percent report constipation as their most frequent symptom, and 30 percent have "mixed" symptoms—perhaps starting off constipated and ending with diarrhea.

IBS is a very specific diagnosis, and we don't put patients with vague complaints into this category anymore. About 80 percent of the information needed to make a diagnosis of IBS comes from the patient's medical history. Symptoms of IBS usually begin in adolescence. The onset of IBS after age 40 is unusual unless it is post-infectious or related to medication. Every patient has a story. If the doctor listens long enough—usually the patient will provide the answer. Sometimes the story sounds very typical of IBS, but sometimes the symptoms do not sound like IBS.

It is important to understand when and how the intestinal problems began. Did the symptoms begin a few weeks after an antibiotic was taken? Or after a food poisoning or gastroenteritis? There is evidence that up to 30 percent of patients will develop IBS-like symptoms after experiencing Salmonella enterocolitis. I specifically ask patients about an antecedent event such as antibiotic use, traveler's diarrhea, a viral gastroenteritis, or food-borne illness. It is widely understood that following gastroenteritis, the brush border of the small intestine is destroyed and lactase is therefore not secreted from the intestinal epithelium. Many doctors tell their patients to avoid lactose and other complex carbohydrates for a few weeks after a severe gastroenteritis to avoid malabsorption, gas, and diarrhea.

Did IBS symptoms begin after a medication change? For example, Fosamax for osteoporosis causes heartburn, GI distress or diarrhea. Medications for high blood pressure, such as the calcium channel blockers, cause constipation. Iron causes constipation and the SSRI antidepressants such as Zoloft, and Prozac can cause nausea and diarrhea. Paxil, Remeron and Effexor on the other hand usually are constipating. Certain classes of drugs including the statin (that is, atorvastatin (Lipitor)), and all NSAIDS (Aleve, Motrin, Aspirin, Bufferin, Excedrin) can cause GI distress especially when taken on an empty stomach. Even the Cox-2 inhibitors (Celebrex), which are actually not pure Cox-2 inhibitors, still can cause GI bleeding and GI distress

There are other causes of IBS symptoms. In some patients a traumatic event, such as rape or physical assault, can trigger IBS.

Birth control pills, hormones, and menopause can all cause gut motility disturbances. Just think of the pregnant state—bloat, heartburn and constipation! Estrogen induces the synthesis of nitric oxide synthetase, which affects GI motility by causing bloating and decreased movement of the intestine. Hormonal causes of IBS should be discussed in patients on a new oral contraceptive or estrogen replacement.

Smoking can cause abdominal pain, cramping, and diarrhea. Smoking in women who are taking oral contraceptive pills is extremely dangerous because combining the two can actually cause blood clots and stroke. A history of eating disorders, anorexia nervosa, or bulimia can also lead to GI dysfunction. These patients often benefit from working with a nutritionist. Lack of sleep and exercise affects GI motility. Therefore, anything that promotes an overall state of well being will help the IBS patient too—from a heart healthy, smoke free diet to swimming, walking and yoga.

"Alarm" symptoms include blood loss, fever, sweats, chills, weight loss, older age of onset (above 30) or a family history of celiac disease, crohns disease or colon cancer. The presence of any alarm symptoms warrant more testing—perhaps colonoscopy, ultrasound, blood work or stool studies for microbiology.

For dietary problems there are some solutions—avoid the trigger foods and there are fewer symptoms. Some patients have food sensitivities that cause gas and bloating. Patients with lactose intolerance develop bloating and gas pains an hour or two after consuming lactose, which is the natural sugar found in dairy products. There are other sugars that are not easily digested—one is called fructose, which is the natural sugar in fruit. Fructose requires a special transporter in the intestine in order to be absorbed. When this transporter is saturated or overused the remaining fructose is left for the bacteria that naturally live in the colon. Products containing high fructose corn syrup, such as Gatroade, sweetened applesauce and Snapple, can lead to abdominal discomfort, distention, and gas. Other triggers for gas pains and bloating are carbonated beverages, such as soda, seltzer, and beer. The gas in the drinks ends up in the intestine causing discomfort, burping, and pain. The artificial sweeteners like sorbitol (in "diet" gums and candies) can also cause gastrointestinal upset. If you are a diabetic and suffer from gastrointestinal upset, try to avoid the "diet" cakes and pies—choose oatmeal or appropriate fruits if you need a snack.

What you will gather from all of the information in this book is that every patient has a different form of illness and perceives and approaches it differently. Each patient is unique but I hope in this book you will find tips that have helped patients similar to yourself. Here are a few examples from the IBS patients I have treated.

IBS medications

Later in this book I discuss treatment options for patients. Sometimes it is key for patients to take medications at an exact time. One patient used a diary to record when she took the medication and the result. Using the diary helped us identify that by eating at the same time every day and having an empty stomach between taking the medications I prescribed and this patient's meals helped her tremendously. We discovered her IBS medicines work best on an empty stomach and then eating anywhere between 45 minutes to an hour after her medicines.

Sugar alcohols

I do tell patients with gas and bloating to avoid sorbitol—an unabsorbable sugar found in sugar-free chocolate, diet gum, candies, and other products. Symptoms due to sorbitol ingestion appear to be related to fermentation of residual carbohydrate in the colon. The other sweetners such as aspartame can cause nausea and other symptoms. The best thing is to avoid sweeteners if you are sensitive to them. I do allow a small amount of honey if patients really need a sweetener.

Supplements

Many calcium supplements (such as oyster shell calcium) are very hard to digest and can cause bloating and constipation. This is because the calcium is not "bioavailable"—instead of being absorbed into the blood it just sits in the intestine and does no good. The supplements that are generally well tolerated include: calcium carbonate (TUMS), chewable calcium (children's preparations or VIACTIVE Calcium with Vitamin D), or calcium powder that you sprinkle on food. Some orange juice is fortified with calcium and the vitamin C in the orange juice helps the absorption. However, it is not clear that calcium is all we thought it was for bone health. Exercise and vitamin D intake may be equally or more important.

Magnesium containing supplements are effective for constipated patients, because the magnesium loosens the stool. Patients with diarrhea should not be given magnesium, because this will exacerbate their problem. Patients with kidney disease also need to be cautious with magnesium intake. Do not take any products or supplements without consulting your physician. Vitamin C is also a natural laxative but all vitmians need to be taken under the supervision of your phyisician. Even "healthy," "natural" products can cause kidney stones, kidney disease or even liver failure. Beware of "detoxifiers" sold on the Internet—that picture of the jelly colon is totally misleading and untrue. There are no toxins accumulating in your colon—actually the lining of the colon (the mucosa) is as clean and pink as the lining of the mouth.

Antibiotics

Tell your doctor very clearly if you took an antibiotic in the months before the IBS symptoms began. Patients who received a recent course of antibiotics are up to three times as likely to report symptoms of irritable bowel syndrome. It may be that antibiotics change the normal bacteria that live in the intestine, or may induce a short-term inflammatory response that causes a sensitive state within the intestine. Antibiotics can even cause a secondary infection called Clostridium difficile ("C diff"). This can cause fever and diarrhea for weeks—rarely it can lead to severe illness or death. C diff is usually treated with metronidazole.

Probiotics

Using a probiotic such as *Saccharomyces boulardii* (Florastor) is helpful in patients with antibiotic associated or post-infectious IBS to treat loose stool, discomfort, and urgency. *Saccharomyces boulardii* can also be taken with an antibiotic to prevent C diff.

Most probiotics cause bloating and may not be useful or worth the money. However, Bifidobacterium (Align) has been studied and shown to improve biochemical and clinical symptoms in IBS patients. Align has been helpful with gas, bloating, urgency, and alternating bowel function (constipation alternating with diarrhea). I recommend patients take Align 20 minutes before lunch. Patients may feel bloated at the beginning of treatment. If the Align is helpful patients can stay on it indefinitely. Some patients take

Align when they are having a bad week—others take it daily. Probiotics cannot be given to people who are immunocompromised (such as chemotherapy patients or HIV patients) because they could become septic.

Hormones

In some patients, GI symptoms can be correlated with starting a new oral contraceptive, pregnancy, menopause, or menses. In these cases, consulting with a gynecologist about changing the hormone replacement or over the counter prescription can be helpful. Using a higher progesterone, lower estrogen pill such as Demulen 1/35 may help in patients who are nauseated and need to gain a little weight.

Diet and lifestyle

Encourage:

- Exercise (exercise helps most patients improve their sense of well-being)
- Sleep (sleep at least 7 to 8 hours per night)
- Soluble fiber (such as oats, beans, barley, bananas, and so on)
- Water (water intake is essential for constipated patients)

Eliminate or discourage:

- Smoking
- Alcohol
- High fat foods, fried foods, and fast foods
- Artificial dweeteners (sorbitol, NutraSweet) if not tolerated well
- High fructose corn syrup
- Carbonated beverages, if not tolerated well
- Gum chewing, if not tolerated well
- MSG, if not tolerated well
- High residue foods such as bell pepper and eggplant skin, if not tolerated
- Raw vegetables such as broccoli or cabbage aren't tolerated well by some (vegetable soup can be enjoyed instead of raw vegetables)

Gas cramps: Anti-spasmodic

The anti-spasmodic I find to be the most effective for my patients is a new preparation of an old medication called hyoscamine. Hyoscamine has been demonstrated to be effective for the pain component of IBS. In my experience Hyoscamine 0.125 mg sublingual (under the tongue) twice a day as needed is effective and well-tolerated in patients with moderate symptoms. I have found the hysoscamine to work within 15 to 30 minutes. Sometimes within a few minutes the patient has relief. At the onset of cramping, at the very beginning of an attack, pop the hyoscamine under the tongue. The sooner the medication gets to the smooth muscle the better—this way the attack, which normally could last for hours, can be abated or minimized. Also, if my patient is on a train, plane, or in a bus and they are afraid of having urgency and diarrhea they can use the hyoscamine, which will give them a few extra minutes and possibly help to avoid an embarrassing episode.

For bloating it is sometimes useful to use a digestive enzyme (Ultrase MT20). These must be taken with food—for example, Ultrase one capsule after 3–4 bites of food and one before the end of the meal. Digestive enzymes are particularly necessary in patients with pancreatic insufficiency, cystic fibrosis or celiac disease—many of these patients also have IBS symptoms.

Treatments for diarrhea

Loperamide slows transit time through the colon and increases intestinal water resorption. The starting dose of Loperamide is 2 mg once a day as needed for diarrhea. We really do not know how long it is safe to use this in IBS. For patients who have post-prandial diarrhea the use of lomotil, immodium, Pamine, immodium or hyoscamine about 30 minutes before a large meal or important social event can improve or avoid symptoms in some patients. It is important to make sure the patient is not infected, impacted, or partially obstructed prior to blocking GI motility. Florastaor is often helpful in a dose of once a day for mild diarrhea (taken before lunch) and twice a day (taken at lunch and dinner) for severe diarrhea. Women with severe diarrhea-IBS can benefit from alosetron (Lotronex). Lotronex is prescribed with a patient-physician agreement. Lotronex cannot be given to patients who had ischemic colitis, blood clots or are risk for a blood clot. Lotronex can be "life saving" for those patients trapped in their homes for fear of having a diarrhea accident.

Digestive enzymes

Pancreatic enzymes such as Ultrase MT 20 are helpful for digestion. Prescription digestive enzymes help patients with celiac disease, cystic fibrosis, pancreatic insufficiency, and maldigestion. The trick is, the lipase in them has to be delivered to the small intestine intact. The coating of the capsule has to be pH dependent to be released in the "alkaline" portion of the duodenum; not in the stomach. Over-the-counter enzymes in general are not effective and are not worth the price. If you need a digestive enzyme, ask your doctor for a prescription. Ultrase is a good brand because it has been provem to have a consistent therapuetic effect and comes with a free supply of ScandShakes (gluten free) or Carnation ready-to-drink (lactose free). Most prescription digestive enzymes have porcine derivatives, and, therefore, if you are allergic to pork, you should not take them.

Fiber therapy

It is essential to differentiate crude fiber (residue) from soluble fiber. Some patients with IBS cannot tolerate residue (bran, bell pepper, eggplant skin) due to increased gas production and discomfort. Soluble fibers (oatmeal, yams, berries) are better tolerated. I rarely prescribe fiber supplements for IBS patients due to side effects of flatulence and discomfort. I do encourage overcooked, mushy vegetables—spinach, escarole, green beans, leeks, turnips, beets and parsnips. Patients who can't tolerate salad but want their veggies do well with a good healthy homemade vegetable soup.

Antibiotic therapy

Rifaximin (Xifaxan) is FDA-approved for the treatment of traveller's diarrhea (Xifaxafan 200 mg 3x/ a day for 3 days). Xifaxan works primarily in the lumen of the GI tract ("gut specific") and has been shown to be helpful in treating flatulence, gas, bloat and diarrhea associated with IBS. Xifaxan is a nonabsorbable antiobiotic (meaning it isn't absorbled into the bloodstream through the stomach and tends to remain intact through the intestinal tract).

I am beginning to investigate the use of Xifaxan for "PMS-IBS." These are patients whose IBS aggravated when PMS comes around. The therapeutic dose varies, but the starting dose is 200 mg, three times a day for three days. For true cases of bacterial overgrowth (characterized by gassiness, foul-smelling gas, cramping, bloating, and sometimes bad breath), we give patients a higher dose of Xifaxan (up to 3 pills 3x a day for 14 days.

What about when IBS seems to be brought on by infections or food poisoning?

Gastroenteritis, rotavirus, or infections such as dysentery, salmonella poisoning, or "Montezuma's revenge" can lead to IBS symptoms. In these cases I treat patients with a low carbohydrate, low lactose, low fiber diets. I also prescribe Xifaxan three times a day for three to 10 days, depending on how severe the episode is. I often follow this with Florastor of Align (250 mg, once a day before lunch).

Alosetron (Lotronex) for diarrhea-IBS

The major advance in the treatment of diarrhea-IBS is the development of Alosetron (Lotronex), which slows motility in the intestine. Alosetron was voluntarily withdrawn from the market in 2000 due to reported complications. The risks of Alosetron (ischemia and constipation) are more common in the elderly institutionalized population, and may be dose related.

Alosetron is only available with a signed consent form, but it can be life-saving for the right patients. The patient and physician each sign a consent form outlining the risks and indications for alosetron. In practice, we prescribe Alosetron 0.5 mg, twice a day as needed. I carefully instruct the patients to drink plenty of water and to hold off on alosetron if they do no not have a bowel movement. I tell my patients to take the alosetron after the first bowel movement of the day—this way patients do not become constipated.

Alosetron is indicated for the treatment of women with severe diarrhea-IBS. I do not recommend Alosetron for patients with unstable angina, heart disease, coronary artery disease, smokers on oral contraceptives or hormones, or any other patient who I think is likely to develop blood clots or pulmonary emboli.

What can I eat, Doctor?

This is meant to be a general guideline and will vary with each patient. If you have celiac disease or sprue, avoid wheat, barley, rye, and their derivatives.

- **Usually tolerated in moderation: soluble fiber:** oatmeal, berries, beets, cooked lentils, legumes, split pea soup, chick peas, peas, carrots, yams, peaches, blueberries, strawberries, papaya, mango, kiwi, organic yogurt, fish, shrimp, rice, pasta, couscous, noodles, pastina, cold egg whites, lentil soup, homemade chicken soup, Udon noodle, Cornflakes, Rice Crispies, Special K, chamomile and herbal teas, nectarines, apricots, plums, watermelon, honey dew, avocado, pears, cantaloupe, avocado, angel food cake, olive oil, broccoli and cauliflower are tolerated best in a puree soup, tender cooked baby spinach, homemade vegetable soup, waffles, pancakes, mashed potatoes, crackers such as low salt wheat thins, rice crackers, unsalted top saltines, baby leaf/red leaf lettuce in small amounts, stewed, tender meat, small pieces of cooked carrots, celery, zucchini with rice, pasta, and couscous.

- **Use Caution:** Citrus, barbeque/charcoal, alcohol, grapes, chocolate, raw broccoli, raw cauliflower, cabbage, cole slaw, cold cuts, iceberg lettuce, popcorn, dairy, caffeine, tomatoes, and lactose

- **Avoid** Crude fiber (residue): Fiber One, Raisin Bran, eggplant skin, bell peppers, cucumber skin, MSG, large seeds, nuts, potato skins, fats, fried foods, carbonated beverages, high fructose corn syrup such as Snapple and Gatorade, garlic, onions, sorbitol, bran, all artificial sweeteners, green tea (nausea)

The symptoms of IBS are common in the United States and affect one in five Americans. Under the umbrella of IBS are complex and diverse disorders that are often confused with celiac sprue, bacterial overgrowth, infectious gastroenteritis, and mild inflammatory bowel disease. The first step to treating IBS is to make an accurate diagnosis of IBS. The next step is to review diet and lifestyle changes with the patient—especially smoking and alcohol cessation and a low fat diet. Then introduce appropriate medications. No matter how you are suffering from IBS symptoms, we will not give up until we have found a few effective treatments to help you!

Christine L. Frissora, MD, FACG, FACP
Associate Professor of Clinical Medicine,
The Weill Medical College of Cornell University

Introduction

I know the label "Irritable Bowel Syndrome" can sound a bit embarrassing (the butt of many a joke, I'm sure) and I know the actual symptoms can be very inconvenient, painful, and debilitating at times (to say the least), but please know two things: (1) You are not alone (one person out of five in the United States adult population is affected by this condition and 60 to 65 percent are of the female persuasion). (2) There are things you can do to make yourself more comfortable and symptom free.

Four things appear to be happening within the body concerning Irritable Bowel Syndrome (IBS):

1. The large intestine appears to move too fast or too slow in sufferers.

2. People with IBS seem to be particularly sensitive to the physical pressure put on the bowel (increasing pain and discomfort).

3. There are often psychosocial factors that can contribute to the intestines reacting strongly—people with IBS often have a greater reactivity to stress, for example.

4. Hormones actually influence the nerves that tell the colon muscles to contract. Changes in certain hormones, such as during the first couple days of your period, can trigger assorted IBS symptoms (painful spasms, gas, constipation, diarrhea).

Q: What does the brain have to do with IBS?

New research from UCLA suggests that women with IBS have a different brain response to abdominal pain than women without the syndrome. Earlier research has shown that in most people the brain can prepare for pain in ways that either inhibit or amplify the pain sensation. The UCLA study suggests that IBS patients cannot turn down the amplifier of the pain response, making them potentially more sensitive to even mild discomfort and pain. [*Journal of Neuroscience*, January 9, 2008]

Good news and bad news...

Being told you have IBS is a good news/bad news situation. The bad news is there is no real cure. The good news is that the condition will never kill you or seriously impair your health. In fact, approximately 60 percent of people with IBS symptoms never seek medical care; these people just live with it. I know because I'm a third-generation irritable bowel sufferer.

So, what can we do? We can at least make ourselves feel more comfortable as we go through life with this syndrome. We can eat a healthful diet (rich in high-fiber foods that our systems tolerate), drink plenty of water, avoid foods that make us feel worse, and find ways to minimize and handle the stress in our daily lives.

But be forewarned: treating IBS is a little like trying to hit a moving target. Not only do IBS symptoms vary from one person to the next, they can also change from week to week in the same person. And when it comes to treatments, different things work for different people. The only way to know what works for you is to try it and see if it helps.

To make things even more complicated, the treatment you try for one symptom can cause a completely new symptom to occur. So with IBS, you definitely want to choose your treatments wisely. That's what this book is about: presenting the possible dietary treatments for IBS (and there is definitely information on the possible medical treatments as well)—many of which have helped IBS sufferers live more comfortable lives. People with IBS who don't seem to respond well to drugs or dietary modification may want to concentrate on the psychological treatments available for IBS. Individual or group psychotherapy, relaxation training, meditation, biofeedback, and hypnosis can all help relieve some symptoms.

You are not alone

IBS has been around for a while. Medical descriptions of IBS can be found from as far back as the late 1800s. After the common cold, IBS accounts for the most missed days of work, and up to 40 percent of all visits to gastroenterologists are related to IBS symptoms. What I find most interesting is that IBS is common across countries that are culturally very different from America, such as Japan, China, and India. IBS affects 5 to 10 percent of the population in both developed and developing countries. So, trust me, you are not alone.

Bowels 101

Whether you are experiencing constipation or diarrhea, knowing how the colon is supposed to work will help you understand what's going on in your body. So let's review the jobs of the large and small intestines, which together are referred to as the bowel or bowels.

Once the stomach has turned food into mush, it releases small amounts of it into the small intestine. The bulk of the digesting and absorbing of the nutrients and calories from the food we eat happens in the small intestine. The pancreas contributes enzymes to help further digest food in general, and bile from the gallbladder and liver helps to break down fat in particular.

What's absorbed? Carbohydrates are broken down into sugars and absorbed. Protein is broken down into amino acids and absorbed. Fat is broken down into fatty acids and glycerol and absorbed. Vitamins and minerals, along with other important nutrients from the food we eat, are also absorbed into the bloodstream in the small intestine. What isn't absorbed? Fiber, for one thing (more on this in other chapters).

The remaining food waste moves to the large intestine, which is also called the colon. The main job of the large intestine is to reabsorb water and salts as the food waste travels through it. This helps form solid stools, which can then theoretically exit the body a couple of days later via the rectum (easily and without discomfort).

These "movements" are controlled by nerves and hormones and by electrical activity in the colon muscle. Muscles in the colon help propel the food waste slowly toward the rectum. "Normal" bowel movements range from three stools a day to as few as three a week. A "normal" movement is one that is formed but not hard, contains no blood, and is passed without cramps or pain.

Sometimes there is too much water for the large intestine to reabsorb, or the food waste travels through the large intestine too quickly, so the intestines don't have a chance to reabsorb enough water, resulting in frequent and/or watery stools (diarrhea). Sometimes there isn't enough water, or the food waste travels too slowly through the large intestine, resulting in infrequent and hard-to-pass stools (constipation).

The mind-body connection

Those of us who have IBS see it as a mostly physical condition, but there is a psychological component to IBS. Some researchers estimate that about half of the patients who seek medical care for

IBS are depressed or anxious. Practitioners have found that the conversion of anxiety into physical symptoms definitely occurs in some of their IBS patients. In recent studies, IBS patients reported lower pain thresholds (they are more uncomfortable than people without IBS with the same amount of induced pain) and more anxiety than women without IBS. Some researchers from UCLA suspect that IBS patients cannot turn down the amplifier of the pain response in their bodies—they then become more sensitive to even mild discomfort.

Think back to when your IBS started. What was going on in your life? The majority of IBS patients report having a very stressful life event just before developing IBS. The event might be a divorce or separation, the death of a spouse or parent, or changing jobs or locations.

Most people will tell you their irritable bowel symptoms are more pronounced when they are stressed. Therefore, if you have an irritable bowel, you must practice stress management and stress reduction as much as possible. Many of us don't even realize what is causing us stress. You might need some professional help to recognize your own personal stressors, such as jumping to conclusions, perfectionism, or seeing problems as catastrophes. Sometimes what we do in an effort to improve matters only makes the stress worse.

Obviously, this is a book about food and IBS, but there are non-food suggestions that you can consider too:

- Practice relaxation strategies (deep breathing, muscle relaxation, imagery, exercise, and so forth).
- Get the rest your body needs.
- Set your priorities realistically.
- Accept, adapt, and learn to let go.
- Work with your healthcare team (ideally a gastroenterologist, a psychologist, and a dietitian) to develop a treatment plan.

If you haven't already done so, please see your physician or a gastroenterologist to identify that you indeed have IBS, because there are many other gastrointestinal diseases that can have similar symptoms.

IBS constipation food guide

If you have IBS constipation, you probably already know how important fiber-rich foods are to your comfort. Making the ADA recommendation to eat 20 to 35 grams of fiber a day your mantra is a great place to start. But in order for a high-fiber eating plan to work its magic, you have to do three things:

1. Reach the higher fiber target (20 to 35 grams of fiber a day) as often as possible.
2. It will work better if you spread out your high-fiber foods throughout the day.
3. Drink plenty of water and other non-caffeinated, non-caloric liquids/beverages throughout the day as well—fiber works better in the intestines if there is plenty of water to go with it. That's one of the reasons why fruits and vegetables are such great fiber choices—they usually come complete with their own water supply!

In the interest of reaching your new 20-to-35-grams-of-fiber-a-day target in the fastest and most painless way possible, here are the five quickest ways to 25 grams of fiber:

1. Get those whole grains!

You can get 4 grams of fiber easily with a serving of whole grains. Here are a few examples:

- 1 to 2 slices of whole grain bread (depending on the brand)
- 1 cup of brown rice

- 1 1/2 to 2 tablespoons of ground flaxseed (depending on the brand)
- 9 Reduced Fat Triscuits and some whole grain cereals

2. Breakfast cereals

Some breakfast cereals contain 5 or more grams of fiber per serving! These can help some people with IBS but can also cause gas. Here are a few examples:

- 1 cup of Raisin Bran = 8 grams of fiber
- 1/2 cup of All-Bran = 10 grams of fiber
- 1 cup of Frosted Shredded Wheat Spoonsize = 5 grams of fiber
- 1 1/4 cups of cooked oatmeal = 5 grams of fiber

Tip: Add your own berries to the cereal!

3. Beans

Beans will boost your fiber totals too! Canned bean products make it easy, and just 1/2 cup can get you to 6 or more grams of fiber in a snap. Here are a few examples:

- 1/2 cup of Ortega Fat Free Refried Beans = 9 grams of fiber
- 1/2 cup of canned kidney beans = 6 grams of fiber
- 1/2 cup of S&W Chili Beans Zesty Sauce = 6 grams of fiber

Keep your serving of beans small until you know how your body handles it. They can cause gas and blating in some people. Beano, a food enzyme supplement that contains alphagalactosidase, helps break down the complex sugars in gas-causing foods and may be helpful for discouraging gas with soy, grains, beans, vegetables, and nuts.

4. Work a few fruits into your day!

- 1 apple = 3.7 grams of fiber
- 1 banana = 2.8 grams of fiber
- 1 pear = 4 grams of fiber
- 1 cup of strawberries = 3.8 grams of fiber
- 1 cup peach slices (fresh or canned in juice) = 2.2 grams of fiber
- 1 cup nectarine slices = 2.5 grams of fiber
- 1 cup cantaloupe or honeydew cubes = 1.4 grams of fiber

5. Work a few veggies into your day!

- 1 cup carrot slices, cooked = 5 grams of fiber
- 1 cup cooked broccoli = 4.5 grams of fiber (can cause gas in some people)
- 1 sweet potato = 4 grams of fiber
- 1 cup cauliflower, cooked = 3 grams of fiber
- 2 cups raw spinach leaves = 3 grams of fiber (can cause gas in some people)

 Easy 7-Layer Bean Dip

Makes 6 big snack servings, although serving of beans is small.

16 ounce can fat-free refried beans

1/2 tsp. chili powder (optional—if tolerated)

1/8 tsp. black pepper (add more to taste, if desired)

1/4 tsp. Tabasco (add more to taste if desired) (optional—if tolerated)

3/4 cup fat-free sour cream

1 cup shredded reduced-fat sharp cheddar cheese

1 cup finely chopped tomatoes

5 green onions, chopped (use if tolerated)

2 ounces chopped black olives (optional)

Suggested dippers: low-fat or reduced-fat tortilla chips, soft flour tortillas or pita bread cut into triangles, or vegetables such as celery sticks, carrot or jicama slices.

1. Add beans to small microwave-safe bowl and heat on high for 2 minutes to warm and soften. Stir in chili powder, black pepper, and pepper sauce to taste. Spread into an 8 × 8-inch baking dish and let cool.

2. Spread sour cream over the beans. Top beans with shredded cheese, then sprinkle chopped tomatoes evenly over the top. Top with green onions and olives, if desired. Refrigerate until needed.

3. Serve with any of the suggested dippers!

Per serving (not including dippers): 145 calories, 10 g protein, 18.5 g carbohydrate, 3 g fat (2 g saturated fat), 10 mg cholesterol, 4 g fiber, 400 mg sodium. Calories from fat: 21 percent.

Cruciferous Au Gratin

Makes 6 side servings.

4 cups cauliflower florets

(Reserve about 2 cups of the coarsely chopped cauliflower stems)

4 cups broccoli florets

2 Tbs. chopped shallots (use if tolerated)

1 Tbs. minced garlic

1 cup golden mushroom canned soup (vegetable or chicken broth can be substituted)

1 cup fat-free half-and-half (low-fat or whole milk can be substituted)

1 to 1 1/2 teaspoons horseradish (or to taste) (use if tolerated)

Salt and freshly ground pepper to taste

1/2 cup packed grated Gruyere cheese (reduced-fat Swiss or Jarlsberg Lite can be substituted)

1. Add cauliflower and broccoli florets to large micro-wave-safe dish with 1/4 cup of water. Cover dish and microwave on high until just tender (about 4 to 6 minutes).

2. Meanwhile, start heating a medium-sized nonstick frying pan over medium heat. Coat the pan with canola cooking spray. Add the coarsely chopped cauliflower stems, shallots, and garlic, and gently sauté until soft (do not brown). Add the golden mush-room soup or vegetable or chicken broth and cook until the stock is almost evaporated. Transfer the mixture to a food processor or blender along with the fat-free half-and-half and pulse until fairly smooth. Add the horseradish, if desired, and season with salt and pepper to taste.

3. Coat a 9-inch pie plate with canola cooking spray. Add the cauliflower and broccoli florets to the dish and pour the half-and-half mixture over the top. Gently toss to blend. Sprinkle the cheese over the top. Bake at 350 degrees for about 15 minutes until golden brown.

Per serving: 115 calories, 10 g protein, 12.7 g carbohydrate, 3.5 g fat (1.9 g saturated fat), 11 mg cholesterol, 3.5 g fiber, 240 mg sodium. Calories from fat: 26 percent.

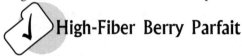 ## High-Fiber Berry Parfait

Makes 1 parfait.

1/2 cup strawberry or berry yogurt (low-fat or light depend-ing on preference)

1/2 cup sliced strawberries

1/2 cup low-fat granola or other whole grain cereal that's tolerated well

Garnish parfait with a small dollop of light whipping cream or light Cool Whip and a whole strawberry, or fan a few slices of strawberries on top (optional).

1. In a 2-cup measuring cup, blend yogurt with sliced strawberries. Spoon half of the mixture into a parfait glass (or similar).

2. Sprinkle half of the whole grain cereal over the yogurt mixture.

3. Top that with the rest of the yogurt mixture and sprinkle the remaining Raisin Bran over the top with a dollop of light whipped cream and a strawberry if desired. Enjoy immediately.

Per parfait: 230 calories, 9 g protein, 50 g carbohydrate, 2 g fat (.9 g saturated fat), 5 mg cholesterol, 5.5 g fiber, 255 mg sodium. Calories from fat: 8 percent.

IBS diarrhea food guide with recipes

Every person with IBS diarrhea has his or her own personal list of foods or types of foods that they may react to in certain amounts. Some of the types of foods that tend to cause problems are greasy, rich, or high-fat meals and snacks.

Fat in food is known to exaggerate the gastrocolonic response, not to mention the fact that fat is harder to digest. You may have already noticed that large amounts of fat eaten in one sitting can cause your bowels to be somewhat "irritable." The key for many people with IBS diarrhea is that fat is better tolerated when eaten in small amounts throughout the day rather than all at once. The other side to eating meals that aren't greasy or high in fat is eating meals that contribute some soluble fiber.

Soluble fiber is the gentler type of fiber that tends to stabilize the intestines. Although soluble fiber is in your intestines, it holds onto water and forms a gel—slowing down the passage of food, which is usually a good thing with IBS diarrhea. Foods high in this type of (soluble) fiber are:

- Psyllium seed and psyllium products.
- Beans (beans contain both soluble and insoluble fiber and can cause gas in some people).
- Oats and oat bran.
- Barley.
- Peeled apples and applesauce.
- Bananas.
- Citrus fruits.
- Carrots.
- Green beans.

Some people with IBS diarrhea have trouble with certain fruits and vegetables. Here is a list of the fruits and vegetables that tend to be well tolerated by the bowels, plus their fiber totals. At the end of the list you will find a few recipes to start you on your way to capitalizing on some of these high-soluble fiber foods and the better tolerated produce gems.

Vegetables (cooked):	Serving Size	Fiber (grams)
Asparagus	1 cup	3.7
Beets, canned, diced	1 cup	3.7
Carrots	1 cup	4
Green or yellow beans	1 cup	4
Green peas	1 cup	8.8
Mushroom pieces, canned	1/2 cup	2
Potato, baked	1 med.	5
Sweet potato, baked	1 med.	3.6

Spinach, boiled	1/2 cup	2.2
Winter squash, baked	1 cup	5.7
Pumpkin, canned	1/2 cup	3.5
Zucchini slices, steamed	1 cup	2.2
acorn squash, baked	1 cup	9
butternut squash, baked	1 cup	6
Fruits (ripe or canned)	Serving Size	Fiber (grams)
Canned peaches in juice	1 cup	3.6
Canned pears in juice	1 cup	3.6
Canned apricots in juice	1 cup	3
Apple (peel the apples if the skin bothers you)	1 large	4.2
Applesauce, unsweetened	1 cup	3
Banana	1 med.	2.3
Grapefruit segments	1 cup	3
Nectarine slices	1 cup	2.2
Kiwi	2	3
Orange sections	1 cup	3.4
Peach slices, peeled	1 cup	3.1
Pear slices	1 cup	4

Cooked foods always go down easier, so if you want to eat a lot of vegetables homemade soup is best; chew all food as well as you can. If you don't have a Crock Pot, get one, because stewed vegetables and meats go down easier than BBQ, broiled, or fried meals. Check out the section, "Get Crocked" in the recipe chapter of this book for a handful of helpful recipes!

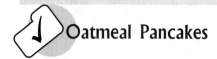

Oatmeal Pancakes

Makes 12 pancakes.

1 1/2 cups quick oats

2 cups low-fat buttermilk

1/2 cup unbleached white flour

1 teaspoon baking soda

1/4 teaspoon salt

1 large egg

1/4 cup egg substitute

1. Add oats and buttermilk to large mixing bowl.
2. Combine flour, baking soda, and salt in 4-cup measure and stir to blend. Add to the oat and buttermilk mixture and beat on low speed until just blended.
3. Add egg and egg substitute and beat on low speed just until blended.
4. Start heating griddle or nonstick skillet over medium heat. When the pan is hot enough, use a 1/4-cup measure to drop batter onto the hot pan or griddle (if the pan or griddle is not "nonstick" coat with canola cooking spray first).
5. Turn pancakes over when the entire tops of the pancakes in pan are covered with bubbles. Cook other side of pancake until nicely brown and cooked throughout. Repeat with the rest of the batter.

Per 3 pancakes (if 12 per recipe): 249 calories, 14 g protein, 38.5 g carbohydrate, 4.5 g fat (1.4 g saturated fat), 57 mg cholesterol, 4 g fiber, 619 mg sodium (485 mg sodium if no added salt). Percent calories from fat: 16 percent.

Peachy Banana Smoothie

Makes 2 smoothies.

2/3 cup orange juice

1 1/3 cups peach slices (frozen unsweetened, ripe, or canned juice and drained)

1 medium banana, sliced

2/3 cup low-fat or light peach yogurt (vanilla can also be used)

2/3 cup nonfat frozen yogurt, light ice cream (with or without sugar as desired)

1. Add all ingredients to your blender or large food processor.
2. Blend on highest speed until smooth, about 10 seconds. Scrape sides of blender and turn on blender for five seconds more.
3. Pour into three glasses and enjoy!

Per smoothie: 250 calories, 8 g protein, 47 g carbohydrate, 3.5 g fat (1.8 g saturated fat), 2 mg cholesterol, 4 g fiber, 80 mg sodium. Calories from fat: 13 percent.

Italian-Style Acorn Squash

Makes 4 servings.

1 medium acorn squash (or other similar winter squash)

1 Tbs. no trans margarine with 8 grams fat per tablespoon

2 Tbs. shredded Parmesan cheese

1/2 tsp. Italian herb blend

1/4 tsp. garlic powder

1. Cut acorn squash in half lengthwise. Add squash, cut side up, to a large microwave-safe baking dish with 1/2 cup water. Cover dish and microwave on high until tender throughout (about 15-20 minutes).

2. Cut each half crosswise several times about 1/2-inch deep and spread margarine evenly over the top.

3. In small dish, blend Parmesan cheese, Italian herbs, and garlic powder. Sprinkle this mixture evenly over the top of each half.

4. Microwave uncovered, on high until cheese starts to melt (about 2 minutes). Cut each half in half to make 4 servings total.

Per serving: 132 calories, 3 g protein, 30 g carbohydrate, 2 g fat (.5 g saturated fat), 1 mg cholesterol, 9 g fiber, 64 mg sodium. Calories from fat: 14 percent.

Chapter 1

Everything You Ever Wanted to Ask a Gastroenterologist

So you think you may have an irritable bowel? Depending on where you live, you may have to wait as long as a few months to see a gastroenterologist to confirm it. And when you do see one, chances are you'll forget to ask a few of your questions. Also, as time goes on, you might think up new questions. That's what this chapter is for.

Q: What is Irritable Bowel Syndrome (IBS) and what are the symptoms?

The "irritable" bowel is more sensitive and reactive than a "regular" bowel. It begins to spasm after only mild stimulation or in situations that a normal bowel would not react to, such as:

- Eating (see tips on changing your eating style in Chapter 4). The simple act of eating causes contractions of the colon, normally causing an urge to have a bowel movement 30 to 60 minutes after a meal. With IBS, the urge can come sooner, along with cramps and diarrhea.

- Distention from gas or other material in the colon (for tips on avoiding gas-producing foods, see Chapters 3 and 4).
- Certain medicines.
- Certain foods (see tips in Chapters 3 and 4).
- Stress, which stimulates colonic spasms in people with IBS.

Some people have diarrhea (or several soft bowel movements) right after they wake up in the morning or right after they eat a meal. IBS symptoms may worsen in the presence of stressors such as travel, big social events, or changes in daily routine. For some, symptoms seem to get worse when they do not eat right or if they eat a big meal.

Q: Will my IBS eventually go away?

Part of the nature of IBS is that it varies from person to person. Generally though, IBS symptoms fluctuate through time. In one study, more than half the IBS patients still had symptoms five years after they were first diagnosed. Some researchers report that almost one-third develop IBS after a bout of the stomach flu or food poisoning. In these cases, the symptoms are usually milder and can diminish during a 3-to-5-year period.

Q: What causes IBS?

IBS continues to mystify the experts. When colons of IBS sufferers are examined, there are no signs of disease. Yet IBS can cause much pain and distress to the people who have it. Researchers are getting closer to the truth, though. They have discovered that the colon muscles of people with IBS begin to spasm after only mild stimulation. Their colons appear to be more sensitive, reacting strongly to events that would not bother most people, such as eating a large or rich meal or having a bit of gas in the colon.

Are you one of the women out there who seems to suffer from IBS-like symptoms only during menstruation? One-third of women who otherwise don't have gastrointestinal (GI) symptoms have them only during their periods. Researchers suspect that reproductive hormones help trigger IBS symptoms, because about half of women with IBS report worsening symptoms—most often diarrhea—during their periods (*American Journal of Gastroenterology* 93[10]: 1867, 1998 and *British Journal of Obstetrics and Gynaecology* 105[12]: 1322-25, 1998).

It is also possible that a lack of hormones could encourage IBS-like symptoms in some women. A recent study suggests that peri- and post-menopausal women have a high prevalence of IBS-like gastrointestinal complaints (*Women's Health* 27[4]: 55–56, 1998).

Experts also suspect that many people have a genetic predisposition to IBS. All I know is that I have a mild form of IBS, my mother has it, and her father had it. Sounds like a genetic link to me! New research also suggests that about one-third of IBS sufferers have a genetic mutation that is also linked to panic disorder.

Although scientists aren't certain why, childhood constipation and colic (as well as childhood physical or sexual abuse) increase the likelihood of developing IBS as an adult.

Q: When would surgery help me?

(answered by Christine Frissora, MD)

Sometimes there are true structural problems in the colon that cause a change in bowel function. If you are a woman or man in a high-power position, doctors may say "it's just stress." But the truth is that stress can exacerbate any problem, including IBS—but it is often not the entire cause of the problem. So how do you know if something needs to be done?

Of course, if there is a family history of colon cancer, bleeding, or a personal history of colon cancer, it may be time for your colonoscopy (yes, again!). If women need to use their finger, "digital manipulation," to defecate, then that is called "vaginal splinting," and it may be due to a structural problem and may improve with surgical intervention. Conversely, if you have given birth or received an episiotomy (the vagina opening is deliberately cut to allow the baby to come out without tearing the opening) and cannot hold stool, and suffer from fecal incontinence (feces or stool or liquid stool leaking into the underwear), then it may be possible that the rectal muscle is torn, severed, or atrophied and needs to be repaired. In this case, you need to see a surgeon who specializes in the rectum.

A warning here: there is no problem that surgery cannot make worse. If you are doing well on your medications and diet, proceed with the appropriate testing and screening but do not seek surgical intervention. Do not try to fix something that you can deal with by changing your diet, or taking simple medications. If you truly need surgery due to a stricture or a rectal tear, you need a very thoughtful, meticulous surgeon.

There are many in the country—the doctor I refer patients to in my New York practice is Dr. Toyoki Sonoda. Dr. Sonoda treats a wide variety of colon and rectal diseases, such as colon and rectal cancer, inflammatory bowel disease, diverticular disease, benign conditions of the anus, and functional problems such as rectal prolapse and incontinence. He has completed specialty training in laparoscopic colon and rectal surgery, and performs laparoscopy for many of these conditions. He can be contacted at (212) 746-6030.

For women with bladder and GYN issues with prolapse I use Lauri Romanzi, MD (212) 935-4343, contact@urogynics.org

Urogynics was founded by Dr. Laurie Romanzi in 1998. Dr. Romanzi and her team bring insight and innovation to the field of women's health. Dr. Romanzi is a clinical professor in the Department of Obstetrics and Gynecology at New York Presbyterian Hospital—Weill Cornell Medical College, and a board certified gynecologist and fellowship-trained specialist in urogynecology and pelvic reconstructive surgery.

Q: Can medicines I take for other things be making my IBS worse?

(answered by Christine Frissora, MD)

Sucralfate, calcium channel blockers, bismuth subsalicylate, and antacids containing aluminum can sometimes aggravate constipation. Other medicines can do the opposite and induce diarrhea. Magnesium-containing antacids, lactulose, and sometimes psyllium and other fermentable fibers used as bulking agents (which can also worsen bloating) may all cause diarrhea.

Q: How do stress and anxiety affect IBS?

Stress may worsen IBS symptoms, plain and simple. Stress stimulates colonic spasm in people with IBS. We don't completely understand why this happens, but we do know that the colon is controlled in part by the nervous system and that the nervous system reacts to stress.

Stress-reduction (relaxation) training or counseling and support help relieve IBS symptoms in some people. But please understand you don't have IBS because you have a psychological problem. Remember, IBS is in large part a result of hypermotility and hypersensitivity of the colon.

One study showed that people with IBS scored higher in measures of anxiety and obsession, but not in measures of phobia, depression, somatic anxiety, and hysteria. The anxiety and obsession are thought to be the consequences, and not the causes, of the IBS symptoms (*Lancet* 340[8833]: 1444–48, 1992).

Q: Which types of psychotherapy might help?

Three types of treatments are yielding some success with IBS patients:

1. **Brief psychodynamic therapy** is conducted one-on-one with a psychiatrist or psychologist for a short time (such as once a week for two months). The goal of this therapy is to explore and identify potential unconscious factors that may be linked to IBS symptoms and to help the patient bring those factors into consciousness to better understand and control them.

2. **Cognitive behavioral therapy** is also performed by a psychiatrist or psychologist in either a group or one-on-one format. The purpose of this therapy is to teach people to cope a little less negatively with life's stressors. IBS sufferers are guided into identifying how they send themselves conscious negative messages. Maybe they take on more blame for situations than they should, or maybe they make things out to be worse than they really are. Patients are often asked to explore what areas of their lives are stressful and how they themselves contribute to the stress with their own perceptions. Repeated therapy sessions enable patients to gradually react more positively to the stressors in their lives—which translates into reduced bowel symptoms.

3. **Hypnosis** teaches people to use imagery to gain control over the muscles in their GI tracts. This can take place in a group or in one-on-one sessions under the direction of a psychiatrist or psychologist with hypnosis experience. Many patients using this method report less pain, bloating, cramping, diarrhea, and constipation.

If you would like to find a psychologist or psychiatrist with experience in treating IBS, the American Psychological Association can direct you to your state associations, which can refer you to a practitioner in your area. Call (800) 964-2000.

Q: Could my symptoms indicate something else?

If there is blood in your stool or if you have been having chills or fever, then you probably have something other than IBS.

A small number of people who think they have IBS could instead be suffering from a new family of disorders caused by hard-to-detect changes in the lining of the large intestine. With these disorders (microscopic colitis, collagenous colitis, and pericrypt eosinophilic enterocolitis), the colon looks normal. But if a bit of the tissue is examined under a microscope, inflammation or scarring can be seen.

Profuse watery diarrhea can be caused by something other than IBS. Frequently, and more often in women, it is actually due to laxative abuse. This is probably far more common than we know because people who abuse laxatives often keep it a secret from their physicians and families. Diarrhea can also be caused by rare, hormone-secreting tumors of the pancreas.

Q: Could I have a food allergy?

Many of the clinical signs typical of intestinal food allergies and intolerance are the same as those that many people experience with Irritable Bowel Syndrome. It is a good idea to find out if you have a food allergy or intolerance. A 1999 study in the *American Journal of Gastroenterology* found that more than 50 percent of the IBS patients studied were sensitized to some food or inhalant without showing any typical clinical signs. Usually the patients were unable to identify the potentially offending foods.

Q: How long does it take for a meal to move through the digestive tract?

Food passes through the esophagus and into the stomach almost immediately. However, it can take as long as three or four hours after a meal before the stomach completely empties into the small intestine. It can take even take longer, depending on the size and fat content of the meal (larger and higher fat meals stay in the stomach longer). The small intestine will take four to six hours to finish digesting a meal and absorbing its contents. It can take two to three days before food waste is finally formed into a stool and emptied from the rectum.

Q: Why do I seem to have several bowel movements first thing in the morning?

When you wake up in the morning, your bowel wakes up too. Normal nerve connections trigger the large intestine to increase its activity (like after meals), particularly first thing in the morning.

Q: Can lack of sleep bring on symptoms in some IBS patients?

Lack of sleep can result in physical or mental stress, which can trigger the IBS symptoms. If you think about it, the gut is at rest during sleep, so it makes sense that daytime activities continue at night if you are awake or tossing and turning.

Q: Can traveling bring on symptoms?

There are many ways that traveling can trigger IBS symptoms, namely the lack of physical activity while traveling long distances, the disruption of routine due to changing time zones, and eating and drinking differently than we normally do. Keeping up with your fiber goals and exercise routine while you travel can help prevent the constipation that frequently results.

Q: Do some IBS patients suffer from stomach-related symptoms during one of their intestinal "attacks"?

The pain of IBS can be anywhere in the abdomen region. Some patients experience nausea, bloating, and other gut symptoms. If there are additional symptoms, such as vomiting, weight loss, signs of anorexia, fever, gastrointestinal bleeding, fever, fecal incontinence, persistent severe pain, or night symptoms, it suggests there is something other than IBS going on.

Top 10 things most likely to be confused with IBS

There are many diseases that have the same symptoms as IBS—gas, bloating, indigestion, flatulence, discomfort, diarrhea, and constipation. The following are the conditions and diseases that are not IBS but can be confused with IBS, according to Christine Frissora, MD.

1. Celiac disease. A genetic, inherited multifactorial condition that results in a lifelong allergy to gluten—barley, wheat, rye, and possibly oats. The treatment is a lifelong strict avoidance of gluten. The Celiac Center led by Dr. Peter Green in New York is among the best in the world.

2. Mild inflammatory bowel disease. Mild ulcerative colitis or Crohn's disease can be missed because they can show up from time to time. If you have a family history of inflammatory bowel disease, weight loss, bloody diarrhea, or fever, tell your doctor.

3. Lymphocytic or microscopic colitis. Characterized by diarrhea and sometimes weight loss. If you have chronic diarrhea, your doctor must do duodenal biopsies to exclude celiac or other causes of malabsorption, and colon biopsies to exclude microscopic or lymphocytic colitis.

4. Blastocystis. This is a parasite one can get anywhere—from take-out food to a dirty bathroom in an airport. There are different treatments, but a low dose of metronidazole, 375 mg twice a day for 7 days, is usually enough.

5. Giardia. This is a parasite from well water or another contaminated supply that can persist for years and cause gas, bloating, and diarrhea.

6. Chronic cholecystitis (gallbladder disease). There may not be gallstones, but if you have had persistent, vague abdominal pain that worsens with eating and fatty

foods, it could have been the gallbladder all this time. Be sure you have an ultrasound—CT scans can miss gallstones.

7. Chronic diverticulitis. There are a few patients that have had recurrent diverticulitis, and the segment of colon is left smouldering and infected. If you have known diverticulosis, severe pain, diarrhea no matter what you do, chills, night sweats, or fever bring this to your doctor's attention immediately.

8. All artificial sweeteners can cause severe nausea, upset stomach, and discomfort.

9. Your supplements can be making you sick. "Natural" health remedies have been known to cause kidney failure, liver failure, and pancreatitis. Do not take any supplement without asking your doctor. In general, with digestive disorders, less is more.

10. Ectopic pregnancy—whether you are on a birth control pill or not, if you have developed bloating, nausea, and abdominal pain, you might be pregnant. Even if you had your period, you could still have an ectopic pregnancy (a pregnancy outside of the uterus).

Dr. Frissora has some final words of advice as you move forward with the rest of this book and with managing and finding relief from your IBS.

Top 9 things you should know if your doctor doesn't

(answered by Christine Frissora, MD)

1. Gallbladder removed?

If you have had your gallbladder removed and in the weeks or months that follow you develop diarrhea, this could be "bile salt diarrhea." It means that the bile drips into the intestine and when it hits the colon can cause diarrhea. The treatment for this is to take something that binds bile acids before you eat, such as carafate (sulcrafate) 1 gram tablets.

2. Calcium supplements and vitamin C.

Calcium supplements that contain magnesium or zinc can cause loose stools. This would be good for someone who is constipated but is not good for someone who has diarrhea.

Vitamin C is a natural laxative and can also cause heartburn, indigestion, and even esophagitis.

3. Proton Pump inhibitors could be triggering your bowels!

Sometimes diarrhea (and possibly abdominal pain) will begin days or weeks after starting a PPI (proton pump inhibitor) and the doctor just doesn't put it together when you go in for help, according to Dr. Frissora. Common PPI medications include Aciphex, Omeprazaole, Prevacid (lansoprazole), Protonix (pantoprazole), and Prilosec, Nexium (esopmepraole). "After you stop the PPI medication, the diarrhea should go away within 7 to 10 days if not sooner," advises Dr. Frissora. The PPI most likely to cause diarrhea is Prevacid (which can be helpful to a constipated patient with heartburn), and the PPI with the seemingly fewest side effects is Protonix. "So if you are constipated and have GERD, ask for Prevacid—it may solve both problems," she says.

If you have GERD, Dr. Frissora suggests losing weight (if obese or overweight) and sticking to a low-heartburn diet. (*Tell Me What to Eat If I Have Acid Reflux* is a great resource for heartburn-free diet and food tips.)

4. All antihistamine medications, including Benadryl, are constipating.

If you are suffering from chronic constipation, consider whether your antihistamine medications might be contributing to it.

5. All antibiotics can cause "C diff."

Clostridium difficile is an infection in the colon that can proliferate after taking an antibiotic. The diarrhea and discomfort can begin days or weeks after the antibiotic is taken. There can be fever, pain, diarrhea, and a foul gassy smell. The treatment options include metronidazole (Flagyl), vancomycin, Florastor, and Questran—for difficult cases these can be used in combination.

6. IBS comes in many shades and varieties.

A thorough medical history, including surgeries, diet, travel, and medications (including birth control pills), is essential to honing in on the correct diagnosis and the proper treatment. Sometimes something as simple as changing from a brand to a generic birth control pill could be enough to trigger bloating, nausea, or discomfort.

7. Artificial sweeteners of all kinds should be avoided.

The alternative sweeteners often used in "sugar-free chocolate," such as sorbitol and mannitol, cause diarrhea and bloating. If you take liquid medications, they may contain artificial sweeteners as well. NutraSweet, Splenda, Equal, and Sweet'N Low can all cause nausea and dyspepsia (upper abdominal discomfort). High fructose corn syrup, a sweetener added to many foods and beverages in America, can cause bloating and diarrhea. Check all labels, especially "light" yogurt—they commonly have artificial sweeteners in them. Yogurts such as Activia (with added probiotics) can actually be too strong for some patients, while it can help others with IBS.

8. Probiotics are not well understood yet.

Some probiotics can cause bloating or nausea. When you swallow a billion bacteria, you can expect gas and bloating. The two I have found most useful are:

- *Saccharomyces boulardii* (Florastor) 250 mg twice a day for diarrhea (taken 1/2 hour before a meal) or to treat or prevent antibiotic-associated diarrhea and "C diff."
- Align can help gas, bloating, and urgency.

Try not to spend a fortune on "natural" remedies though. A lot of them do not have any safety or efficacy data to support their use. Probiotics cannot be given to immunocompromised people— that means if you have cancer, AIDS, or are taking prednisone, you should not take probiotics.

9. The scoop on antidepressants.

Sadly, most antidepressants, although good for relieving pain, can cause fatigue, weight gain, and sexual dysfunction. The tricyclics (amitriptyline, Elavil, desipramine) are constipating and the SSRIs (Zoloft, Prozac) are more likely to cause diarrhea. Having said that, if I have a thin, anxious person with diarrhea and insomnia, I may give desipramine 10 mg at night. If I have a thin, bloat-pain patient, then I use Celexa 10 mg at night. If the patient exercises and cuts carbs, there should be no significant weight gain. At these low doses, side effects are rare.

Wellbutrin is good for smoking cessation and does not cause weight gain (also sold as Zyban for smoking cessation). It is an "upper," and if you are anxious, Wellbutrin can make anxiety worse. It can also cause seizures. Having said that, for an overweight, lethargic smoker, a little Wellbutrin in the morning can be helpful. Wellbutrin usually promotes weight loss and smoking cessation. Its role in IBS is less clear. None of these antidepressants are FDA approved for IBS per se. There are studies and medical experts, though, who have used them for years to the benefit of their patients. The trick is finding the best antidepressant for each particular patient considering their overall gastrointestinal and psychological health.

Chapter 2

Main Symptoms of Irritable Bowel Syndrome

What Irritable Bowel Syndrome means to me could be, and probably is, quite different from what it means to you. Each of us experiences different symptoms with varying severity. Certainly though, specific symptoms do tend to be associated with Irritable Bowel Syndrome. These symptoms are listed and discussed in this chapter.

Abdominal pain

A typical pattern in IBS is the beginning of pain, soon followed by a somewhat formed bowel movement and relief (albeit temporary) of the pain. But shortly after this, the bowel spasms (causing pain), resulting in more watery bowel movements over several hours. The pain many people experience with IBS feel is often in the lower part of the abdomen, below the belly button, although some feel it throughout the abdomen. The pain often gets worse 60 to 90 minutes after meals. Research has shown that people with IBS have a lower pain threshold for gastrointestinal tract distension than people without IBS. However, their tolerance of other painful stimuli is at least equal to that of healthy controls. Therefore, it is suggested that this pain may be due to a higher sensitivity of the bowel in people with IBS.

Irregular pattern of defecation at least 25 percent of the time

This is a fancy way of saying there is a disturbance in the frequency, form (hard vs. loose/watery), or passage (straining, urgency, feeling of incomplete evacuation) of your stools some of the time. You are actually more likely to see episodes of irregular bowel function alternating with periods of normal bowel with an "irritable" bowel than you are with an "inflamed" or diseased bowel. You might have a regular bowel movement every day, except every fourth week or so when your bowel movements are either more constipated or looser. Or you might only experience intestinal problems first thing in the morning or late at night.

Some people suffer mainly from constipation, others primarily from loose stools, and some suffer from both.

Constipation-predominant IBS

Constipation-predominant IBS often starts in adolescence and may result from excessive colon contractions, which lead to stool dehydration (hard, stiff stools). People with this type of IBS seem to improve with a high-fiber eating plan. The goal is to consume around 30 grams of fiber a day, so many people have to use fiber supplements.

If you increase your fiber too fast, you might suffer from bloating and gas. To prevent this, you can use warm tap water enemas along with the fiber supplement. Also, your physician may add osmotic laxatives (glycerine suppositories, for example) or stool softeners if fiber alone isn't doing the trick. The use of stimulant laxatives is definitely discouraged.

Diarrhea-predominant IBS

Maybe you wouldn't describe what you have as diarrhea; maybe the term "loose stools" is a little more accurate. Or maybe you have diarrhea sometimes and soft stools most of the time. Loose stools in IBS are usually of small volume but frequent. Having to go in the early morning or after meals, as well as stress-related urgency, is also common in people who experience this symptom.

I know that, for me, the early morning sometimes offers a certain challenge. I usually have to go to the bathroom two or three times within the first hour after I wake up. This wouldn't be so bad if I didn't also have to make breakfast, pack two lunch boxes, get two girls ready for school, feed the dog, and let her out. I'm often in the middle of making toast when all of a sudden I have to scurry around the corner to the closest bathroom. Not because I have diarrhea, just because I have urgent stools.

This type of IBS may have something to do with what's going on inside the intestinal space (not the wall or muscle of the intestines). Carbohydrates, bile acids, short-chain fatty acids, or food allergens might be inside the intestines causing problems as they move through. Maybe they aren't being digested properly. Maybe they are being broken down by bacteria or causing water to move into the intestinal space. Soluble fiber may actually improve diarrhea for some by helping hold onto water when it is in the intestines (more on soluble fiber in Chapters 3 and 4).

Mucus in the stool

Half of all IBS patients report mucus (without blood) in their stools. If you see blood mixed with mucus in the stool, this is not IBS; it is more likely to be colitis (inflammation of the colon). I know it is a bit alarming to find mucus in your stool, but mucus is normally produced by the intestine to serve as a lubricant. It's just that some people with IBS might be producing extra amounts.

Abdominal bloating or swelling

Abdominal bloating or swelling is a common symptom of IBS, especially if you are constipated. The bloating usually worsens as the day goes on and improves after sleeping. If you are able to better manage your constipation or diarrhea, abdominal bloating and swelling may well subside.

The feeling of incomplete emptying of the rectum

Most people who suffer from this symptom empty their rectums completely when they go to the bathroom. This symptom is a result of an oversensitive rectum, which causes a "false alarm."

Gas attacks

For some people with IBS, it isn't the gas that bothers them as much as it is the abdominal pain and bloating that tend to come with it. Reducing the amount of gassy foods in your diet will help relieve abdominal pain, gas, and bloating.

Many gas-producing foods contain carbohydrates that are not completely digested in the small intestine. By the time they get to the end of the large intestine, bacteria (normally present in the intestines) have digested these carbohydrates and produced gas as a breakdown by-product.

However, some people with IBS may have a specific disturbance in bacterial fermentation and colonic gas production. Studies have found that gas production in the colon (hydrogen gas in particular) is, indeed, greater in people with IBS than the rest of the population.

Symptoms occur or intensify during menstruation

For many women, IBS symptoms seem to be worse during their periods. Right before your period (if you can plan ahead) and certainly during it, it is especially important to avoid trigger foods or stressors that seem to bring on or aggravate bowel symptoms.

Beyond the bowels: Common IBS symptoms in other parts of the body

- Studies have shown that some people with IBS also have heartburn.
- Another symptom is sleep disturbance, which often aggravates IBS symptoms.

- Fatigue is a common complaint with IBS patients. Fatigue can be a result of disturbed sleep or exhausting periods of diarrhea, or it may indicate clinical depression or other serious psychological problems.
- Bladder or urinary problems are also associated with IBS. It may be that an irritable bowel causes a generalized sensitivity of the smooth muscle that lines the bowel and bladder.
- Non-cardiac chest pain (a sharp or dull ache in the central chest that cannot be ascribed to heart disease) sometimes also occurs in people with IBS.
- Nausea, bloating, or pain in the upper abdomen may be present.
- Migraine headaches have been linked to IBS. Smooth muscle, which lines the intestines, also lines the blood vessels that cause the throbbing effect of migraines. But beyond this, the mystery of why migraines and IBS are associated has not been solved.
- Painful intercourse has been noted by some women, perhaps due to an increased sensitivity of the other organs in the pelvis.
- Some people with IBS also suffer from fibromyalgia, a condition in which muscle and tendons have increased sensitivity and areas of tenderness and pain. With fibromyalgia, intense and persistent pain can be felt in the abdominal wall muscles.

Chapter 3

Everything You Ever Wanted to Ask Your Dietitian About IBS

A big part of treating and managing IBS involves what you eat, how much you eat, and where you eat. Certain foods and nutrients can help you, and others can make your symptoms worse. This book is designed to help you discover which foods to emphasize and which not to touch with a 10-foot chopstick.

Remember while reading this chapter that IBS is a very individual disorder; you may have to try several treatments until you find one that works for you.

Even if your IBS is particularly affected by stress, you still need to know about the link between foods and IBS, because stressful times are when you need to pay the closest attention to your diet. Limiting your personal food triggers will help minimize the symptoms during the difficult time.

Q: What foods are good for diarrhea?

Have you heard of the BRAT diet before? (It includes bananas, rice, applesauce, and toast.) Well, I call it the BRATY diet now—I added yogurt with active cultures if tolerated. Dr. Frissora recommends the following to her patients:

- Bananas, white rice, rice crackers, rice milk, and white meat chicken.
- Pedialyte for rehydration (not Gatorade, which is high in fructose).
- Isomilk DF (binding infant formula with calories).
- *Saccharomyces boulardii* (Florastor), the most effective probiotic for diarrhea—one a day.
- White rice and candy corn (this is very binding).

Q: What foods are good for constipation?

When this is the issue, Dr. Frissora recommends the following to her patients:

- Five servings a day of foods such as oatmeal, berries, pears, peaches, plums, papayas, mangoes, kiwis, raisins, prunes or prune juice, chickpeas, carrots, celery, snap peas, snow peas, peas, and green or yellow beans.
- Five glasses of water or herbal decaffeinated tea—more if you can.
- Avoid foods and supplements, such as white rice, that improve diarrhea.
- Overcooked spinach or green beans with a little olive oil and vitamin C (no more than 1 gram with dinner) are natural laxatives.

Q: What are the foods/drinks that may cause bloating or stomach distress?

Dr. Frissora has found quite a few specific foods that seem to cause bloating or stomach distress in some of her patients.

- Most probiotics cause bloating (*Saccharomyces boulardii* does not).
- Cheese (especially larger amounts) can bring on gas and bloating in some people.

- Bran fiber can cause foul-smelling gas and bloating in many patients. If you think you are one of these people, try avoiding bran or products with added bran and see if it helps. Notorious products that cause gas are: Raisin Bran and Fiber One, and Grape Nuts cereals. Dr. Frissora's patients say, "I was trying to be healthy!" It may be healthy, but it's gassy too. Try egg whites or oatmeal with berries for breakfast instead, advises Dr. Frissora.

- Nuts can be hard to digest for some people, sometimes causing abdominal pain. If you don't have a problem with nuts, try organic or natural nut butters.

- All carbonated beverages, such as beer, soda, and seltzer, can cause gas and bloating because some have fructose and other potentially offending ingredients.

- All alternative sweeteners (sorbitol and other sugar alcohols, Splenda, Equal, Sweet'N Lo, aspartame, and NutraSweet).

- Fructose corn syrup (used in all sorts of foods and beverages so check the ingredient label).

- Zone bars, and some other brands of power bars can cause bloating.

- Green tea can cause nausea in some. You can try making it iced or more diluted than usual and see if this helps.

- Onions and garlic.

- MSG (monosodium glutamate), particularly for people who have a sensitivity to it.

Q: Which changes in my diet might help relieve my symptoms?

There are foods to choose and foods to lose. People with mild, constipation-predominant IBS may benefit from an increase in soluble and insoluble fiber. Fiber can help because it improves the way the intestines work in some people. It may reduce bloating, pain, and other symptoms. Some people find more improvement with soluble-fiber foods; I happen to be one of them. I consider soluble fiber a gentler fiber; it forms a gel with water while in your intestines. You'll find a list of soluble-fiber food sources and supplements in Chapter 4.

To know which foods to lose, you will have to keep an FFS journal—of food, feelings, and symptoms—for a few weeks (more on this in Chapter 4). However, you may already have ideas about which foods aggravate your symptoms. You may find your symptoms worsen after you eat foods very high in fat or caffeine. Products containing sorbitol (an artificial sweetener used in sugar-free candy and gum) and antacids that contain magnesium can cause diarrhea. Beans, peas, cabbage, and some fruits give many people gas. Milk products can cause trouble in people with lactose intolerance or lactose maldigestion. Alcohol and high-sugar foods trigger symptoms for some.

In general, Dr. Frissora has noticed that cooked foods seem to go down easier. So, if you want to eat a lot of vegetables, homemade soup is a great way to go. Chew all the foods you eat as well as you can before swallowing, and dust off that slow cooker, because stewed vegetables and meats go down easier than food that's been grilled, broiled, or fried.

Q: How do I know what my trigger foods are?

If you aren't sure which foods might be triggering your IBS symptoms, start by keeping an FFS journal for a couple of weeks. Play detective and try to find the links between the food, eating patterns, and symptoms. This is a very important step, which I'll discuss in greater detail in Chapter 4.

Q: What should you do if you suspect that a particular food is causing you problems?

Totally avoid the suspected food for at least two weeks. Then try a small amount of it, either with foods you know you tolerate well or by itself. If you don't notice any symptoms, give it another day just to be sure. If you do notice symptoms, avoid it for another week and try it again (at a time when getting the symptoms wouldn't be terribly inconvenient) just to be sure.

Q: Should I consider trying a wheat-free and/or dairy-free diet?

Many gastroenterologists suggest this to their patients, particularly the ones with diarrhea-dominant IBS, to see if it brings some relief. The "placebo effect" could be responsible for some of the perceived benefits, but it's probably worth a try, especially if dairy or wheat comes up in the food diary (more on the food diary in Chapter 4) as a potential trigger.

Q: Why do some foods seem to bring on IBS?

It is all too easy to say "avoid these foods" or "these are bad foods for people with IBS and these are the good foods." The truth is, it just isn't that simple. Sometimes it isn't so much what you eat, but how much you eat, or how many trigger foods you eat in one meal or one day—or how much stress you're under while you eat. (Irritable bowel symptoms are more pronounced when you are stressed.) With IBS, you may have to look beyond the specific foods to see the patterns, keeping in mind that the effects of trigger foods can often be unpredictable.

When looking for patterns, ask yourself:

- How much of the symptom-provoking food did you eat at one time?
- Did you eat two or more symptom-provoking foods at once?
- Did you eat one or more symptom-provoking foods at one meal and then one or more at the next meal?

Q: What do I need to know about vitamins if I have IBS?

We know now that the key components and vitamins in foods have synergy with other components in foods, so it is usually best to get your nutrients through food. For a book about the revolutionary science of food synergy, check out *Food Synergy* (Rodale, 2008). But, if you have IBS and you want to take vitamins, this is what Dr. Frissora advises her patients:

- If you have a sensitive stomach and need iron, use chewable children's vitamins such as Flintstones with iron.
- If you do not menstruate (because of menopause or a hysterectomy) do not take any vitamins with iron—usually the "silver" multivitamins will match this need.
- If you are constipated and are menstruating, use CitraNatal DHA after dinner.
- If you have diarrhea and are menstruating, use Prenate after dinner.

Q: Do I need to cut any foods out of my diet if diarrhea is one of my main symptoms?

You could try cutting out lactose-rich dairy products and sorbitol-containing diet products (such as sugar-free gum and mints) to see if the diarrhea improves. Other foods that tend to aggravate diarrhea are salads, bran products, beans, broccoli and related vegetables, apples, and excessive fat, alcohol, and caffeine.

Q: Why do I develop symptoms after eating in restaurants or eating a big meal?

Having recently gotten a puppy, I am well aware that dogs need to relieve themselves, like clockwork, after a meal. The simple act of eating normally causes the muscles in the colon to contract. In people without IBS this might cause an urge to go to the bathroom 30 to 60 minutes after a meal. But in people with IBS, this feeling is more urgent and may come sooner—and with cramps and diarrhea. Does that mean you should eat as few meals a day as possible? Actually you should do the opposite—eat many smaller-sized meals.

You see, the greater the number of calories in the meal (especially from fat) the stronger the post-meal response tends to be. Food fat, from any source—animal or vegetable—is a strong stimulant of colon contractions. Generally, when we eat large, high-calorie meals, they also tend to be high in fat, delivering a double whammy to our intestines.

Eating out is particularly challenging for many people with IBS. Restaurant servings are usually large, and the food is typically rich in fat and calories. For practical tips on eating out with IBS, check out Chapter 7.

Q: Which foods or drinks, even in small amounts, bring on symptoms in some people with IBS?

Certain food substances, such as caffeine, alcohol, sorbitol, other sugar alcohols, fructose, and fat, have gut effects even in healthy people. Their effects will be exaggerated in someone with IBS. If people without IBS have an uncomfortable reaction to a big bowl of baked beans, imagine what it could do to someone with IBS. Now, many experts hesitate to make lists of food triggers because they don't want to create a fear of certain foods; I don't either. But if you talk with people who have lived with IBS for years, they usually can name several foods or food substances that spell trouble for them. Those in the following list came up in several research and anecdotal sources, and have been known to give non-IBS sufferers trouble when eaten in large or small amounts.

Fructose (the natural sugar found in fruits and berries) has been shown to increase abdominal distress in people with IBS. It is possible that the bacteria in the large intestine are breaking down the fructose that was not completely absorbed in the small intestine, resulting in gas, bloating, and/or diarrhea.

Soft drinks containing large amounts of sugar (about 8 teaspoons per 12-ounce can) can wreak intestinal havoc in some people with IBS. Diarrhea is the main effect brought on by the high amount of sugar and possibly the caffeine. Cutting down to no more than one eight-ounce glass on occasion might do the trick.

Sugar alcohols (sorbitol, mannitol, maltitol, xylitol, isomalt, etc.) Sorbitol and other sugar alcohols can be found naturally in some fruits and plants, and they are used as low-calorie sweeteners in various food products because they aren't easily digested. This group of sugar substitutes is particularly helpful to people with diabetes because only a portion is digested and absorbed. And the part that is absorbed through the intestinal tract is absorbed slowly, so there is little rise in blood sugar and little need for insulin.

Because these sugar alternatives aren't easily digested, they have been known to produce gas, bloating, cramping, and diarrhea. The part of the sugar alcohol that *isn't* digested or absorbed goes through the intestinal tract and starts to ferment and attract water. This creates discomfort ranging from gas to diarrhea, depending on the amount consumed and each person's tolerance. The American Dietetic Association advises that more than 50 grams of sorbitol or 20 grams of mannitol per day can cause diarrhea. You can see the total amount of sugar alcohol in a serving of each sugar-free product by reading the nutrition information label.

Olestra (a calorie-free fat substitute made from vegetable oils and sugar) is marketed under the brand name Olean and is used, so far, to make reduced-fat potato chips and crackers. Olestra is not digested or absorbed in the intestines and exits the body—and therein lies the problem. It can exit rather quickly in some people and bring on gas, bloating, diarrhea, and abdominal pain. You may be able to eat only small amounts of products containing Olestra.

Caffeine is an intestinal stimulant that can worsen cramps and diarrhea, so some gastroenterologists suggest that their IBS patients be aware of this and possibly limit their caffeine consumption.

Chocolate, which does contain some caffeine and is obviously high in fat, has been linked to diarrhea and is listed in some references as something to be limited or avoided by people with IBS.

As for me personally, rarely is there a day when I don't have a little bite of chocolate. It is quite possibly the only food I actually crave. You can keep your chips, french fries, candy, and ice cream—all my body asks for is a bit of chocolate in the middle of the day. So believe me, it is with great pain that I list chocolate as a potential trigger food. I don't think it is a trigger for me personally, but then I only have a couple of bites a day (the equivalent of two chocolate Hershey Kisses). Maybe if I had a whole chocolate bar, I would notice an effect.

One expert has noted that the main gut reaction to chocolate is heartburn, because it weakens the lower esophageal sphincter. Perhaps chocolate gives some people trouble because they tend to eat it in large quantities. A dietitian I spoke with remarked that some of her patients appear to be very sensitive to it. So I asked two of the dietitians I interviewed whether people seem to tolerate small amounts of chocolate (such as two Hershey Kisses), as opposed to an entire chocolate bar. One said they probably could, and the other said that small amounts appear to be fine most of the time.

Q: Which fruits and vegetables tend to be well tolerated by the bowels?

There are some general rules of thumb you can follow that can help make fruits and vegetables easier for your body to handle. *Vegetables should be cooked* to reduce potential gas production, and *fruits should be canned* (in juice or light syrup) or *eaten ripe* when the fruit and skin are soft. For specific suggestions, refer to the following list:

Vegetables to try (cooked):

- asparagus*
- pumpkin*
- potatoes*
- carrots*
- green or yellow beans
- green peas

- mushrooms
- beets
- zucchini
- sweet potatoes*
- spinach*
- winter squash*

Fruits to try:

- canned fruit
- peeled apples
- applesauce
- soft, ripe bananas
- grapefruit

- nectarines
- kiwi
- orange/orange juice*
- peaches
- pears

*high in vitamin A (carotene), vitamin C, and/or folate (folic acid)

Q: Which foods are particularly helpful when you are having an IBS episode?

The BRAT diet, prescribed by pediatricians for children recovering from diarrhea, can help. BRAT stands for Bananas, Rice, Applesauce, and Toast. Most people with diarrhea also benefit from other bland foods, such as boiled or poached eggs, crackers, and gelatin.

Getting enough water or other fluids is crucial in order to prevent dehydration from diarrhea. Signs of dehydration include a decrease in the need to urinate, dark or light brown urine, sunken eyeballs, rapid pulse, vomiting, constant thirst, drowsiness, and even unconsciousness.

Q: If I lower the fat in my favorite foods, will I be able to tolerate them better?

Many people I spoke with said yes. Fat in food is known to exaggerate the gastrocolonic response, so greasy or high-fat foods can be problematic for some people with IBS. But that doesn't mean you have to banish your favorite foods forever. Reduced-fat pizza and ice cream, and light (but delicious) recipes for foods such as lasagna and oven fried chicken, might fit into your food plan very nicely.

Q: What is it about my eating style that might be aggravating my IBS?

Some symptoms of IBS can be linked to *how* you eat more than to *what* you eat. Consider the following questions and then ask yourself whether you can modify your behavior.

- Do you eat too quickly? If you do, you might be eating a lot at one time, because it is harder to be aware of how much you are eating, how your body feels, and whether you are satisfied.

- Do you go to fast-food chains often? If you like going to fast-food restaurants, you might just need to change what you order. Fast food is typically high in fat, which can cause indigestion, abdominal pain, and even diarrhea in some people. Choosing items that are lower in fat often helps most people. But it is possible that something other than the amount of fat (such as preservatives) is aggravating your symptoms.

- Do you skip meals or eat a lot of food one day and very little the next? This type of eating style can encourage irritable bowel symptoms such as bloating, abdominal pain, and irregular bowel movements. It is also particularly likely to cause gas.

- Are you a junk-food junkie? Junk food (chips, cheese puffs, and candy bars) is high in fat and calories, but offers very little in the way of nutrition. These popular snacks can be hard to digest, leading to indigestion, gas, diarrhea, and abdominal pain.

- Do you sometimes overeat? People with irritable bowels often become highly symptomatic after eating large amounts. You may have noticed that during or after holidays, when many of us eat much more than our stomachs can possibly hold, you end up with indigestion, bloating, abdominal pain, and/or nausea. This could very well be because you tend to overeat at holiday meals (which also tend to be high in fat).

Q: Is there anything I can add to my diet to discourage IBS symptoms?

Not getting enough fiber or water on a daily basis can aggravate some IBS symptoms. There is evidence that at least 30 grams of fiber a day will improve constipation and some other symptoms.

People with IBS-constipation are a lot more likely to meet this fiber goal in the future, because we have extra motivation to do it. If getting enough fiber helps alleviate some of our IBS symptoms, you better believe we are going to make sure we get enough fiber. I notice the difference when I don't get enough fiber.

High-fiber diets can keep the colon slightly distended, which is actually a good thing, because it is thought to help prevent spasms. Soluble fiber, which dissolves in water and keeps water in the stools, helps prevent hard, difficult-to-pass stools. I personally think of soluble fiber as the gentler fiber. While in your intestines, it holds on to water and forms a gel (slowing down the passage of food—usually a good thing with IBS sufferers), then moves toward the end of the intestines in an orderly fashion.

But what about bran? Bran is an insoluble fiber that does not dissolve in water. Some trials report an improvement in constipation with bran. In sufficient amounts, bran is supposed to soften stools and prevent straining during elimination. However, one study found that 55 percent of patients reported that bran made their IBS worse *(Lancet* 344 [8914]:39, 1994). Besides wheat bran, you can get insoluble fiber by eating unpeeled fruits, whole grains, and most vegetables.

Don't forget to drink plenty of water and increase your fiber slowly to avoid the gas and bloating that can accompany a quick increase in fiber. (Even if this does happen, it will dissipate after a few weeks as your body adjusts to the change.)

Q: Which foods can I eat that are high in gentler soluble fiber?

Here is a table listing the foods highest in soluble fiber. Hopefully you'll find plenty of foods that you personally know and love!

Food	Soluble Fiber (g)	Total Fiber (g)	Calories	Protein
Top 20 Soluble Fiber Foods				
Passion fruit, 1 cup	12.3	25	229	5
Guava, 1 cup	4.5	9	112	4
Navy beans, 1/2 cup	2.8	9.5	127	8
Refried beans, 1/2 cup	2.5	6	110	7
Cranberry beans, 1/2 cup	3.4	9	120	8
Cherrios, 1 1/2 cups	2.9	4.5	165	5
Red kidney beans, 1/2 cup	2.7	7	112	8
French beans, 1/2 cup	2.6	8	114	6
Split green peas, 1 cup	2.5	8	117	8
Asian pears, 1	2.4	4	239	1

Food	Soluble Fiber (g)	Total Fiber (g)	Calories	Protein
Top 20 Soluble Fiber Foods				
Life cereal, plain, 1 1/2 cups	2.3	4	239	6
Rye crisp bread crackers, 2 ounces	2.1	9	207	5
Pinto beans, 1/2 cup	2.1	6	103	6
Black beans, 1/2 cup	2.1	8	113	8
Orange, medium, 1	2.1	3	62	1
Pink grapefruit, 1	2.1	3	91	1
Parsnip, slices, 1 cup	2	7	100	2
Oats, rolled, 1/2 cup	2	4	150	5
Mung beans, 1/4 cup	2	9	179	12
Savoy cabbage, 1 cup	2	4	35	3
Other Sources of Soluble Fiber				
Baby lima beans, 1/2 cup	1.9	7	115	7
Brussels sprouts, 1 cup	1.9	4	56	4
Grape Nuts, 1 1/2 cups	1.8	5	212	6
Roman beans, 1/2 cup	1.7	8	108	7
Persimmon, Japanese, 1	1.7	6	118	1
Mango slices, 1 cup	1.7	3	107	1
Kiwi, 2	1.7	5	93	2
Blackberries, 1 cup	1.7	7	90	2
White beans, 1/2 cup	1.6	9	124	1.6
Pumpernickel, 2 slices	1.6	5	130	1.6
Oat bran, 1/4 cup	1.5	5	58	4

Food	Soluble Fiber (g)	Total Fiber (g)	Calories	Protein
Other Sources of Soluble Fiber				
Flaxseed, ground, 2 Tbs.	1.5	4	86	3
Wheaties, 1 1/2 cups	1.5	5	165	5
Pear, fresh, 1	1.5	7	133	1
Apricots, dried, 1/4 cup	1.4	2	78	1
Triticale, 1/4 cup	1.4	9	161	6
Turnip cubes, 1 cup	1.4	3	34	1
English muffin, 1	1.3	4	134	6
Cornmeal, yellow, 1/4 cup	1.3	2	110	2
Lentils, 1/2 cup	1.3	8	115	9
Garbanzo beans, 1/2 cup	1.3	5	142	6
Prunes, dried, 1/4 cup	1.3	3	104	1
Peaches, dried, 1/4 cup	1.3	3	96	3
Yams, baked cubes, 1 cup	1.3	3	176	3
Rye flour, dark, 1/4 cup	1.2	7	104	7
Peas, green, 1/2 cup	1.2	4	67	4
Collard greens, 1/2 cup	1.2	3	25	2
Great northern beans, 1/2 cup	1.1	6	104	7
Broad beans, 1/2 cup	1.1	5	91	7
Fava beans, 1/2 cup	1.1	5	94	7
Hazelnuts, dried, 1/4 cup	1.1	3	21	2
Beets, cooked, 1 cup	1.1	3	75	3
Acorn squash, 1 cup	1.1	9	115	2
Peach slices, 1 cup	1.1	3	109	2

Food	Soluble Fiber (g)	Total Fiber (g)	Calories	Protein
Other Sources of Soluble Fiber				
Sunflower seeds, 1/4 cup	1	3	186	6
Barley, pearled, 1/2 cup	1	3	97	2
Bulgur wheat, 1/2 cup	1	4	76	3
Pecan halves, 1/4 cup	1	3	187	3
Miso, 2 Tbs.	1	2	68	4
Whole wheat pasta, cooked, 1 cup	1	4	174	8
Wheat Chex, 1 1/2 cups	1	5	162	5
Artichoke hearts, 1/2 cup	1	7	45	2
Carrot slices, cooked, 1 cup	1	3	28	1

Q: Are probiotics helpful?

Probiotics represent some "good" bacteria (live microbial food substances) that may help restore balance among the microflora on your intestinal walls—which is key to maintaining normally functioning bowels. Probiotics are normally found in fermented dairy products, such as yogurt, acidophilus milk, kefir, and in supplement form. These helpful live cultures are able to survive the trip through the stomach and small intestine, and it's in the colon (or large intestine) where they mostly work their magic. There are two specific organisms that showed positive results in recent studies, so look for these specific names on the ingredient list: *Lactobacillus plantarum* and *Bifidobacterium breve*. Dr. Frissora recommends the probiotic, *Saccharomyces boulardii* (Florastor), for people with diarrhea.

Q: Are there any herbs that might help my symptoms?

There are some natural anti-spasmodics out there. Fresh mint leaves, for example, when brewed into a strong tea, can help some people.

Q: How is lactose intolerance related to IBS?

The common symptoms of lactose intolerance are nausea, cramps, bloating, gas, and diarrhea. So you can see how easy it would be to confuse lactose intolerance for IBS and vice versa. The lactose intolerance symptoms will arise anywhere from 30 minutes to two hours after eating or drinking something containing lactose, the sugar in milk.

Lactose is normally broken down into smaller sugars, which are then absorbed in the small intestine. People who are lactose intolerant do not digest lactose well and do not produce enough lactase, the enzyme that breaks down the lactose. Without enough lactase, some of the lactose isn't being broken down and absorbed. This leftover lactose ends up in the large intestine, where it has no choice but to interact with bacteria, resulting in the production of short-chain fatty acids and—what else—gas (mostly hydrogen and carbon dioxide).

If gas wasn't enough, lactose-intolerant people also end up with diarrhea, because lactose, which shouldn't be in the large intestine, attracts water. Extra water in the intestines makes for watery stools. The combination of gas and watery stools is often described as "explosive diarrhea" (that conjures up some undesirable images, doesn't it?).

Between the ages of 5 and 14, many people in America and other parts of the world seem to experience a genetically programmed reduction in lactase synthesis to about 10 percent of the activity they had in infancy. About 25 percent to 30 percent of the U.S. adult population has low lactase activity and could be described as having lactose maldigestion. Certain ethnic groups are more likely to develop it though, with as many as 75 percent of

African-Americans and Native Americans and 90 percent of Asian-Americans being lactose-deficient. It is least common among people of northern European descent.

Similar to IBS, the degree of lactose intolerance varies from person to person. Millions of people suffer from lactose intolerance and don't realize it. And many people think they are lactose-intolerant and are really not. Mildly lactose-intolerant people, for example, may only experience a little extra gas or slight diarrhea when they eat or drink a little too much lactose.

For people with lactose intolerance, there is a rule of thumb to keep in mind: The more lactose you consume, the more severe the symptoms (depending on your particular lactose threshold/tolerance level). Many people with lactose intolerance can handle a small amount of lactose. They can often consume the equivalent of up to two cups of milk a day, as long as the milk is taken in two doses, spaced many hours apart, and consumed with other foods.

If you think you might have a problem digesting lactose:

- **Find out for sure whether you are lactose intolerant.** You can do this with one of two fairly simple tests at your doctor's office. In the hydrogen breath test, patients drink a high-lactose liquid and their breath is analyzed at regular intervals. It works because undigested lactose in the colon is fermented by bacteria, producing hydrogen. The hydrogen travels through the bloodstream to the lungs and is exhaled. Another test is the stool acidity test, which measures the amount of acid in a stool sample. It works because undigested lactose fermented by bacteria in the colon creates lactic acid and other short-chain fatty acids, which can be measured in the stool.

- **Find out how much lactose you can comfortably consume.** How much dairy can you handle at one time, and how many times a day can your body manage it without symptoms? Unfortunately the only way to answer this is through trial and error.

- Start with small amounts of dairy and work your way up.

- Pay attention to the amount of lactose, rather than the amount of dairy products you are eating or drinking, because some dairy products have much less lactose than others.

- Don't consume dairy products by themselves. Have them with other foods.

- **Experiment with lactase tablets** to see if they help you. There are several products available; look for them in your local pharmacy. Just one little Lactaid caplet, for example, works quickly to help you easily and comfortably digest the lactose your body can't quite handle. Just take a caplet with your first bite of dairy foods. You can use it every day, with every meal, if you like.

Q: How come I used to be able to drink milk?

Are you wondering if you weren't lactose intolerant before, why are you now? Certain illnesses can create a lactase deficiency later in your life. This sudden deficiency, coupled with an already declining level of lactase (as we age), can give us a type of lactose intolerance. What type of illness? Scientists suggest that certain infections can change the ecology of the GI tract.

Q: How much lactose is in there?

Many people can manage low-lactose dairy foods, such as ice cream and aged cheeses, but not other dairy products. Some people are perfectly fine with a serving of yogurt, even though it contains about 12 grams of lactose, because the bacterial cultures used in making yogurt produce lactase.

Here's a rule of thumb on dairy and lactose that will leave some people jumping for joy: The higher the fat content of a dairy product, the lower the lactose level tends to be. Rich ice cream tends to be better tolerated than light ice cream or ice milk, and whole milk is usually better tolerated than low-fat and skim milk. By the way, some IBS sufferers say they tolerate chocolate milk (the only kind of milk you'll ever see me drinking) better than plain milk. (The mechanism by which cocoa helps lactose digestion is not yet known.)

	Serving Size	Lactose (g)
Milk (whole)	8 ounces	11.4
Milk (1% or 2%)	8 ounces	11.7
Milk (skim)	8 ounces	11.9
Yogurt (plain)	8 ounces	12
Ice cream/ice milk	8 ounces	5–7
Sour cream	4 ounces	4
Processed cheese	1 ounce	2
Hard cheese	1 ounce	1
Butter	1 teaspoon	trace

Hidden lactose

People with a very low tolerance for lactose sometimes need to avoid food products that contain small amounts of lactose, such as:

- Bread and bread products.
- Cakes, brownies, and cookies.
- Processed breakfast cereals.
- Instant potatoes, soups, and breakfast drinks.
- Margarine.

- Lunch meats (except for kosher ones).
- Salad dressings.
- Candies and snack foods.
- Mixes for pancakes, biscuits, and cookies.

Avoid products containing whey, curds, milk by-products, dry milk solids, nonfat dry milk powder, and, of course, milk. Be aware that 20 percent of prescription drugs and about 6 percent of over-the-counter medicines contain some lactose.

Q: Is it possible I cured my IBS when I eliminated a certain food from my diet?

It's more likely that you had a food sensitivity or intolerance to that food than IBS if you feel you "cured" your IBS, because there isn't a cure. This type of condition continues throughout your life.

Q: Do certain foods make my IBS symptoms worse?

Yes, they certainly do. The tricky part is that the troublesome foods tend to be rather individualized. There are certain foods that seem to be problematic for a lot of IBS sufferers though (and you'll be hearing a lot more about them). Another helpful tip that applies to all IBS sufferers is avoiding large meals. Large meals overload the digestive and intestinal tract and can cause a lot of discomfort and quick trouble for many. Smaller meals are often much easier on the intestinal tract.

Q: Which type of fiber is best if I have IBS constipation?

Fiber can be very helpful for people with IBS constipation, but you need to experiment with caution. Basically, it's important to work with your doctor on types of fiber and fiber products and supplements, because you don't want to make your situation worse. Soluble fiber (psyllium products) has been effective, and some people have found wheat bran (soluble fiber) does relieve bloating and constipation, but it can make things worse for others. The safest way to go about trying a high-fiber diet and/or supplements is to:

- Do it under a doctor's care.
- Increase your fiber gradually.
- Drink plenty of water and other fluids to help your body handle the increase in fiber.

Q: Are there certain foods that seem to aggravate IBS for many people?

The following foods and beverages can be problematic for people with a hypersensitive bowel (IBS), but can even trigger unpleasant intestinal symptoms in people who don't have IBS:

- Greasy or fatty foods.
- Sugar alcohols (such as sorbitol, maltitol, and others) are used as alternative sweeteners in sugar-free chocolate, some gums, and hard candy, and are not absorbed and cause big trouble for some people.
- Caffeine (how much causes trouble and at what time of day is the worst depends on each person).
- Alcohol (how much causes trouble and at what time of day is the worst depends on each person).
- Foods with a lot of high fructose corn syrup.
- Dairy products (if there is some lactose intolerance) and sometimes due to the fat if using high fat dairy products in larger amounts.
- Gas producing vegetables (beans, cabbage family or cruciferous veggies). If these cause trouble for you, try smaller servings and using the slow cooker.

Q: When it comes time to choose margarine for toast or baking, what should I buy?

I suggest, for general health reasons, that people switch to canola oil and olive oil in recipes and use less than usually called for whenever possible. These oils are more likely to contribute the smarter fatty acids and less of the worst fatty acids.

However, there are certain situations, in the kitchen or on the table, when you want a margarine product (buttering toast, making cookie dough, whipping up a light frosting, and so on).

When margarine is needed, I suggest choosing one that has less fat (8 grams of fat per tablespoon works well). Most of these products have water as the second ingredient and hopefully liquid canola oil, soybean, or olive oil as the first ingredient. If you are using margarine with more water than this or less fat grams per tablespoon, it may not function well in the pan or in your recipes.

Even within this guideline, there are some better choices out there:

- Try to find margarine with the least amount of saturated fat and zero trans fat.
- Try to find margarine with omega-3s if possible (if canola oil is used or if fortified with omega-3s).
- You can choose margarine with plant sterols added too. This is preferable particularly if you or someone in your family has elevated blood cholesterol.

Q: Where does this leave butter?

I use whipped butter for certain recipes that call for browning butter (margarine doesn't brown; only butter does, due to its impurities). I always use less butter than called for in the original recipe. When you use whipped butter, you are also getting less fat per tablespoon (around 7 grams per tablespoon compared to 12 grams of fat per tablespoon with stick margarine or butter).

Chapter 4

The 10 Food Steps to Freedom

We know that irritable bowel symptoms range from constipation to diarrhea, and symptom severity varies from person to person. We know that different food strategies help different people. We also know many studies have failed to show that particular foods cause IBS. But does that mean there isn't anything we can do to help manage our symptoms? Of course not.

There are foods that do affect intestinal activity, even in people with normal bowels. It makes sense that these effects will be exaggerated in someone with IBS, whose intestines may react more strongly to various stimuli. The basic strategy here is to minimize negative food effects and keep our bowels healthy. We can work to slow down the very fast bowel and to gently speed up the very slow bowel. Try these steps for at least six weeks, as it can take that long for your body to adjust and respond. These food steps might be enough to help manage milder conditions, in which the symptoms are occasional, stress related, or caused by too much food or drink.

Because everyone's irritable bowel syndrome is unique to him or her, consider these three keys to managing your symptoms:

1. Understand the links between diet, stress, and your symptoms.
2. Match possible management strategies to your symptoms.
3. Pay close attention to which strategies seem to help which symptoms.

The first food step to freedom involves keys one and three. The other food steps will arm you with diet strategies that can help you manage your symptoms. Some food steps may be more helpful to you than others, so focus on the food steps that work for you.

Food Step 1: Keep an FFS Diary (Food, Feelings, and Symptoms)

Food Step

Keep a log of what you eat and drink, your feelings, and your irritable bowel symptoms for a couple of weeks. The information will help you (and perhaps your medical team) not only identify foods and eating patterns that trigger your symptoms but also find solutions that help. According to Dr. Frissora, food and lifestyle diaries are also helpful to pick up non-food-related problems that could trigger IBS symptoms such as sleep patterns, smoking, alcohol, and exercise.

About feelings and stress

- General feelings and worries can influence how you experience your irritable bowel symptoms.
- Stress may not affect the bowel until several days after you experience it.
- Stress may not affect the bowel to the same degree and in the same way each time.
- In this modern, busy life, we have become so used to stress that we have trouble identifying it. Ask yourself what was stressful about your day and if there are any events or feelings you want to note.

Writing the diary entry

Choose a set time each day to write in your FFS diary. You might prefer the end of the day, when things tend to be calm and you have a bit of time to yourself. You can think back over the day and write down what you ate and drank, how you felt, whether you were stressed, and any IBS symptoms you experienced, including time of day and severity. Dr. Frissora's patients report their smoking, gum-chewing, intake of carbonated beverages, fructose-containing food, and alcohol. She also asks patients to record when each medication was started in relation to the patient's symptoms. (You can find a blank entry form on page 94.)

Food Step 2: Eat high-fiber foods (as tolerated)

Food
Step

Notice that this food step doesn't say "eat fiber," it says "eat high-fiber foods." We know that both types of fiber benefit our bodies in many ways. But there are other nutrients and phytochemicals in high-fiber foods that help fight cancer and heart disease as well. You'll read more about some of these later in the chapter.

In order for a high-fiber eating plan to work its magic, you have to follow it every day. Also, it will work better if you spread your high-fiber foods throughout the day.

Don't try to make up for all the fiber you've been missing in a matter of hours. Start with small quantities of high-fiber foods and slowly increase up to 25 to 30 grams a day.

One more thing: You shouldn't increase your fiber without increasing fiber's partner—water. Drink plenty of liquids (preferably those without caffeine, alcohol, or a lot of sugar). See Food Step 3 for details.

Remember how I've mentioned quite a few times already that every IBS patient is a little different, even within the specific types of IBS? Well, the same goes for how well fiber helps the body.

Studies have found conflicting results on how helpful certain fiber supplements (such as Citrucel) or wheat bran have been for people with IBS. For example, in most research wheat bran seemed to help relieve constipation and bloating, but it may actually worsen symptoms in some people too.

The best way to go about this is to experiment with fiber and see what helps you personally, but do so under a physician's guidance. Don't forget to increase the amount of fiber slowly (throughout many weeks) and to drink plenty of water along with it!

Fiber's role in the intestines

Fiber is made up of complex carbohydrates that are not digestible by human enzymes. It is one of the last components of a meal to leave the stomach. The body holds on to the fiber in the stomach as long as it can, so that the fiber doesn't interfere with the digestion/absorption of the other food components that are going on further down in the intestines.

When the fiber makes it down to the large intestine, bacterial enzymes normally present in the intestines try to break some of it down. Nutrients from this breakdown are absolutely crucial for the normal health of the cells that line the large intestine. (Gas can also be a by-product of this bacterial breakdown of fiber.)

If you suffer from periodic constipation or diarrhea

It doesn't come as a surprise that people with irritable bowel syndrome who battle periodic constipation benefit from high-fiber diets. When we think of constipation, we think of needing roughage. But actually, if you suffer from the diarrhea type of IBS, a gentle fiber supplement and bulking agent, such as psyllium, may be helpful too. It can add many grams of fiber quickly and painlessly.

There are several psyllium products on the market, but you should be aware that they can produce bloating in some people. I have been using Perdiem, a psyllium supplement, before bed and have found it helps minimize my morning symptoms without any bloating or other side effects. For those who do have problems with psyllium, there are synthetic bulking agents (polycarbophil or methylcellulose) that are supposed to be less likely to produce bloating.

Start with half the suggested dosage and increase throughout the next few days, until you reach the full dose. For example, the Perdiem instructions suggest that adults and children 12 years old and older take 1 to 2 rounded teaspoons once or twice a day. Work up to this dosage by starting with a rounded half teaspoon once or twice a day. After a couple of days, increase to 1 teaspoon once or twice a day, and after a couple more days, increase to 1 1/2 teaspoons once or twice a day. Finally, a few days later, increase to 2 teaspoons once or twice a day.

6 fiber tips for people with irritable bowels:

1. Try to eat about three servings of whole grains or whole-grain products (breads, rolls, crackers, muffins, or cereal) each day. Throughout recent years, scientists have credited most of whole grains' health attributes to their fiber. We also now know the nutrients and phytochemicals found in whole grains play a role in preventing cancer and heart disease. Whole grains contain:

   - Lignans—which appear to function as antioxidants, preventing cellular changes that can lead to cancer.
   - Flavonoids—which may reduce the risk of heart disease.
   - Tocotrienols—which are powerful antioxidants that help prevent the formation of dangerous cholesterol.
   - Saponins—which may bind with cholesterol in the digestive tract and escort it out of the body.

- Vitamin E—which is an important antioxidant and has been linked to reducing the risk of heart disease and some cancers.

- Minerals (zinc, selenium, copper, iron, manganese, and magnesium)—which help protect body cells against damage from oxygen.

2. Find out which type of fiber works best for you—soluble or insoluble. (Oatmeal and barley are rich in soluble fiber; other whole grains are rich in insoluble fiber.) Both fibers benefit our bodies, but in different ways (see box in Chapter 3), so getting a combination is generally best for the public at large. But what about people with IBS? Although some experts recommend focusing on insoluble fiber for irritable bowels, the soluble fiber grains (oats, barley, psyllium) are still well tolerated and fine for most people with IBS. In fact, some people fare better with soluble fiber than insoluble.

3. Don't have most of your fiber all at once—spread your fiber foods/supplements throughout the day.

4. Focus on getting fruits and vegetables (which have fiber and important nutrients) that are better tolerated and tend not to form gas in people with IBS. For example, cooked yams, parsnips, turnips, carrots, and green and yellow beans (for a list, see Chapters 2 and 3).

5. Drink eight or more eight-ounce glasses of water every day (see Food Step 3 for details).

6. Give it time. It takes the intestinal tract up to six weeks to adapt to a new, higher fiber food plan. However, your intestines might never adjust to some foods, such as cabbage or certain beans.

Food Step 3: Drink eight or more 8-oz. glasses of water

Food Step

Caffeine-free liquids, such as juice, milk, and herbal tea, can count toward two of the eight glasses of water per day. The rest has got to be good, old-fashioned H_2O. Healthy bowels need plenty of water to be able to do their job right. And if you are following Food Step 2 and eating plenty of fiber, drinking more water is even more essential—the two go hand in hand.

I know it is difficult to drink all those glasses of water. I have to work on it every day. These tricks have helped me:

- I bring some water with me when I step into the car.
- I try to drink a glass of water or cup of tea right when I wake up (it's one of the first things I do) and another one right before I go to bed. That's two glasses right there.
- I like to drink "fun water" every day. I treat myself to a glass of water with ice and a slice of lemon, or a glass of flavored (unsweetened) mineral water (it comes in flavors such as lime, lemon, and cola berry).
- Find a decaffeinated green or black tea that you *really* like. Then make a batch of iced tea to keep in the refrigerator. I enjoy peach-ginger and tropical flavored green tea, iced or hot!

Food Step 4: Limit caffeine

Food Step

Coffee is an example of a drink that you may tolerate only in small amounts or not at all. Why? Coffee contains caffeine, and caffeine stimulates the muscles in the digestive tract. That morning cup of Joe gives your intestines a jolt along with your brain. You may have noticed how it seems to wake up your large intestine about 30 to 60 minutes after you drink it. Caffeine also stimulates the kidneys, causing them to release more water into the bladder than needed. This diuretic effect certainly seems to counteract everything in Food Step 3, doesn't it?

The number-one source of caffeine in the American diet is coffee. Second in line are colas and other soft drinks. How do you get around this? Drink primarily decaffeinated coffee to minimize muscle stimulation and dehydration from coffee. Be aware, though, that you still may suffer stomach pain or heartburn from it.

I like my coffee just as much as the next gal, but as far back as I can remember, I've been drinking decaf. I noticed way back when that when I drank coffee I had trouble sleeping and would get jittery, weak, and light-headed within an hour. Not exactly the effect I was looking for. I personally don't depend on coffee for a pick-me-up, I just happen to love its flavor, so decaf easily satisfies me.

The best-known source of caffeine is coffee, of course, but you might not expect to find a similar amount (or more) of caffeine in prescription or over-the-counter medications, energy drinks, soda, or even gym and ice cream.

Beverage	**Caffeine (mg)**
Coffee, 6 ounces	
Automatic percolated	70–140
Filter drip	110–180
Instant, regular	60–90
Instant, decaffeinated	0–6
Tea, 6 ounces	
Made weak	20–25
Made strong	80–110
Cola (12-ounce can)	20–60

Food Step

Food Step 5: Avoid high-fat meals and snacks

I'm afraid IBS is yet another reason not to eat lots of fatty foods. Fat in food is known to exaggerate the gastrocolonic response. Fat is harder to digest, so the higher the fat content of your meal, the longer it tends to stay in the stomach before moving on to the intestines.

You may have already noticed that large amounts of fat eaten in one meal can cause your bowel to be somewhat irritable. Does that mean you need to go fat-free all the way and treat fat as the enemy? Absolutely not. You can have your fat and eat it too—just don't go overboard. Remember that fat is better tolerated when eaten in small amounts throughout the day rather than all at once. You are going to have to work out what this means to you personally in terms of your food choices and your symptoms.

I have personally noticed that I can be quite comfortable eating half an order of tempura (Japanese battered and fried shrimp and vegetables). But if I eat the entire order, I'm done for. And if I go to a restaurant, I can do well if I order just one dish that is high in fat. But if I also eat a rich dessert and perhaps a high-fat appetizer or side dish, troubles are sure to follow.

What about making high-fat favorite foods lower in fat? Does that make them easier on the bowels? Clinicians tell me that for many people the answer is yes. My own experience has shown that this is true for me. So, for example, a lower-fat spaghetti made with very lean ground beef and mild seasonings will probably go down better than spaghetti made with greasy, spicy sausage. Or you might find that you feel fine after eating an extra-lean burger made at home with oven-baked steak fries, but that you definitely do not after eating a bacon cheeseburger and fries at a diner. Keep this in mind when you look over your FFS diary.

You will find ideas to help you avoid high-fat meals in Chapter 6 (supermarket tips) and Chapter 7 (tips for eating out). For ideas when cooking at home, take a look at the following information and the recipes in Chapter 5.

Q: How low can you go?

How much fat can you cut and still maintain the taste and texture of the original recipe? Each recipe has an *ideal fat threshold* (the minimum amount of oil, butter, margarine, or shortening), needed to produce a food that tastes like its fat-laden original. If you go below this ideal amount of fat, or if you don't use a suitable fat replacement, you won't be happy with the results. I've been "lightening" recipes for 15 years and I've written six cookbooks, so trust me on this. Throughout the years, I have developed ideal fat thresholds and fat replacements for different types of recipes.

My favorite fat replacements

Ideal fat replacements are the fat-free or lower-fat ingredients best used to replace fat removed from a recipe. The following ingredients constitute my fat replacement arsenal. All of these foods add flavor and moisture with little or no fat. I believe there is an ideal fat replacement for each recipe. For example, I might use lemon yogurt as a fat replacement in corn bread and maple syrup as a fat replacement when making chicken sausages. I tend to use light sour cream as a fat replacement in brownies, but I prefer to use fat-free cream cheese as a fat replacement in cookies. I might use coffee liqueur as a fat replacement in a graham cracker pie crust.

Buttermilk

Buttermilk makes a nice fat replacement in certain recipes because it is thick and adds a distinctive, pleasantly sour flavor. I always buy the smallest container, because it tends to spoil rather quickly.

Chocolate syrup

While it may sound high in fat, chocolate syrup is virtually fat free and contains about 40 to 50 calories per tablespoon. Use it instead of some of the oil or melted butter in cakes or brownies. You can reduce the granulated sugar called for in the recipe to compensate for the added sweetness from the chocolate syrup.

Cream cheese (fat-free or light)

Fat-free cream cheese makes a nice replacement for butter or shortening when the thick richness of fat is crucial, as is the case with cookies, rich cakes, frostings, pie crusts, and biscuits.

Flavored low-fat yogurt

I like to use flavored low-fat yogurt as a fat replacement for oil in quick breads and sometimes in cakes and coffee cakes. You can have a lot of fun with the different flavors; try coffee or vanilla in a chocolate cake and lemon or orange in a spice cake.

Light or fat-free sour cream

I use light or fat-free sour cream as a fat replacement for butter or shortening in cakes and brownies (and sometimes dressings, gravies, and such).

Lemon juice

I like to use lemon juice in place of most of the oil in marinades or salad dressings, and even in cakes or quick breads, because it adds a lot of flavor, even in small amounts.

Fruits and fruit purees

I use crushed fruit, such as crushed pineapple, or fruit purees, such as applesauce or apple butter, when their flavors complement the other ingredients in a particular recipe. For example, I'll use crushed pineapple in place of some of the oil in a carrot cake, or apple butter instead of half the butter in a spice or coffee cake.

Fat-free, reduced-fat, or light mayonnaise

There are times when I might use reduced-fat mayonnaise in place of fats or oil, such as when I need something that will coat a food or help a crumb coating adhere. I also use it for thickening, for example, in a reduced-fat creamy salad dressing.

Maple syrup

I have used maple syrup instead of lard in chicken sausages and in place of oil in spice cakes, quick breads, and certain types of cookies.

Molasses

Substitute molasses for some meat marinades or sauces. Molasses can also be used as a replacement for some of the butter or oil in certain quick breads, coffee cakes, and spice cookies.

Corn syrup

You can reduce the amount of sugar called for in baking recipes and then replace some of the fat with corn syrup. There's something about the chemical structure of corn syrup that makes it hold on to its moisture in a baked product longer. It releases moisture slowly, through time, into the food.

Food Step 6: Avoid trouble spices

Some people with IBS are not able to tolerate hot sauce, spicy barbecue sauce, or foods that contain:

- chili powder
- curry
- hot chili peppers
- ginger
- garlic

You may tolerate these spices in small amounts, or it could be that not all of them cause problems for you. You might do just fine with curry, ginger, and garlic, but have trouble with chili peppers or chili powder.

Take heart, though—there are ways to add flavor and spice to your dishes without precipitating IBS symptoms. Use the herbs and spices that tend not to be problematic, such as basil, oregano, thyme, and rosemary.

Food Step 7: Avoid overdoing alcohol

Alcohol stimulates the digestive tract by getting digestive juices flowing, so it can cause heartburn, stomach pain, and diarrhea. People with IBS (and, frankly, everyone else) would be wise to keep alcohol intake moderate:

- One drink a day for women.
- No more than two drinks a day for men.

Instead of having an alcoholic drink at the end of the day, at a restaurant, or at a party, you can:

1. Order a fancy drink without the alcohol, such as a virgin daiquiri, margarita, or Bloody Mary.

2. Enjoy many of the great-tasting non-alcoholic beers that are now available. The less-expensive brands are Sharp's and O'Doul's, and imported brands such as Kaliber and Clausthaler.

3. Have a coffee drink (without alcohol or caffeine when possible).

4. Ask the bartender for club soda or sparkling mineral water with a wedge of lemon or lime.

5. Enjoy an iced or hot tea (decaffeinated when possible).

6. Order hot chocolate for a change, especially during the winter.

Food Step 8: Avoid gassy foods

Food
Step

For some people with IBS, it isn't the gas that bothers them as much as it is the abdominal pain and bloating that tends to come with it. Reducing the amount of gassy foods in your diet may help relieve the symptoms of abdominal pain, gas, and bloating.

Many gassy foods contain carbohydrates, which are not completely digested in the small intestine. By the time they get to the end of the large intestine, bacteria (normally present in the intestines) has digested these carbohydrates and produced gas as a breakdown by-product. Which foods are we talking about (as if you don't already know)? Certain fruits and vegetables, dried beans and peas (and dairy for people who are lactose intolerant), and any of the sugar alcohols are particular offenders.

The following vegetables can cause trouble even when they are cooked: lentils, dried peas, and beans, including black-eyed peas, navy beans, kidney beans, split peas, and lima beans.

The following fruits can cause trouble in some people: apples (with peel), honeydew, melon, avocados, prunes, cantaloupe, and watermelon. Other food/drinks that may cause trouble are beer, seeds (sesame, poppy, sunflower, flaxseed), hard-boiled eggs, soft drinks, nuts, wheat germ, popcorn, and spices (chili powder, garlic, hot sauce, curry, ginger, spicy BBQ sauce).

Some people with IBS may have a specific disturbance in bacterial fermentation and colonic gas production. Studies have found that gas production in the colon, particularly of hydrogen gas, is indeed greater in people with IBS compared to controls. One recent study put IBS gas sufferers on a standard exclusion diet. Beef and dairy were excluded (and replaced by soy products), cereals other than rice were excluded, and yeast, citrus fruits, and caffeinated drinks were restricted. The researchers concluded that gas production and symptoms were reduced (*Lancet* 352[9135]:1187, 1998).

Food Step 9: Eat smaller, more frequent meals

Large meals can bring on cramping and diarrhea in people with IBS. Post-meal exacerbation of pain and other gastrointestinal symptoms were seen in about half of a sample of patients with IBS (*American Journal of Medicine* 107[5A]:33S-40S, 1999).

By eating smaller meals and portions, but eating more often, we reduce the intestinal load at any one time. You are pacing the intestines, not giving them more than they can handle at any one time. When you think of it that way, it makes sense, doesn't it? Don't even think about skipping meals. Your bowel likes routine. It wants you to eat regular meals, which means not skipping meals if you can help it.

Easier said than done

Our society is based on three meals a day (with dinner traditionally being the largest), so if you eat out often, you will find this food step particularly difficult. Restaurants tend to serve large portions and that's all there is to it. It requires extra diligence at restaurants to eat only half your meal and save the rest for later (or order less to begin with). If you are having spaghetti, for example, you could eat the salad and half your entrée, then have the bread and the rest of your spaghetti later or the next day. I'm not saying it isn't going to be difficult, but it can be done. If it helps minimize your symptoms, it is well worth it.

Food Step 10: Exercise!

Food
Step

Exercise can be therapeutic for people with IBS. Certainly exercise helps those who tend to have bouts of constipation. This is because exercise is another intestinal stimulant. Moving around and using muscles seems to help get things moving in your gastrointestinal (GI) tract. It can also be helpful for the people with other IBS symptoms, because exercise is a powerful stress reducer. By exercising, you are helping to reduce the stress that could contribute to an IBS flare-up.

You might find that your body prefers to exercise at a certain time of day. Perhaps first thing in the morning works for you and seems to minimize constipation. Or, if your bowel is most active first thing in the morning, exercising later on might suit you better. Experiment with different times.

Another option is to exercise in short spurts throughout the day. For example, you could walk your dog in the morning and then ride your stationary bike while you watch a half-hour show in the evening. Or, if you work in an office, you can walk the long way from your car, the subway, or the bus station to your office and take the stairs a few times during the day. Then, maybe do a little something at home in the evening. Often we are most limited by our lifestyles and work schedules, so do what you can.

If you haven't been exercising on a regular basis, getting started is the hardest part. Once you get going though, and you start feeling the difference (more energy, less constipation, better sleep), it's easier to keep it up. If you are a self-described couch potato, then maybe riding a stationary bike while you watch TV is a good place to start. I personally find an hour goes by quickly when I'm watching one of my favorite shows atop my comfortable stationary bike. One of the keys to exercise success is finding types of exercise you actually enjoy doing that also fit into your lifestyle. Do this and you will be much more likely to stick to it.

Q: How much fiber?

The National Cancer Institute and the U.S. Food and Drug Administration recommend between 25 and 30 grams of fiber per day.

FFS Diary

Day_____

Time	Foods/Drink	Symptoms/Severity	Stress/Feelings

Notes

Possible food triggers

Q: Never heard of psyllium?

Psyllium is a grain grown in India. Its seeds happen to be high in soluble fiber. Since the early 1900s, American pharmaceutical companies have been making over-the-counter bulk-formers from psyllium seed.

Warning: Some people have an allergic reaction to psyllium, ranging from stuffy noses, itchy eyes, coughing, and wheezing to (very rarely) anaphylactic shock. So start with very small amounts until you know you are not allergic.

Q: Is there an alternative to psyllium?

If bloating is a major problem, Dr. Walter Coyle, Gastroenterology PRogram Director for the Scripps Clinic, uses Citrucel (methylcellulose), which does not usually cause bloating, as an alternative to psyllium.

Q: What does each type of fiber do for you?

Fiber does a whole lot more for our bodies than just keeping things moving.

Soluble fiber: Oats, beans, psyllium, and some fruits and vegetables (carrots, apples, citrus). Lowers cholesterol; helps reduce risk of diabetes.

Insoluble fiber: Husks of whole grains, wheat bran, and stalks and peels of fruits and vegetables. May help reduce risk of colorectal cancer, diverticular disease, varicose veins, hemorrhoids, and obesity.

Fiber also helps us eat less by lowering insulin, an appetite stimulant, and by making us feel full.

Ideal fat thresholds and fat replacements for different types of recipes

Recipe	Fat Threshold	Fat Replacements
Biscuits	4 tablespoons shortening for every 2 cups flour.	Fat-free cream cheese, nonfat or light sour cream.
Cake mixes	No additional fat is needed because most mixes already have 4 grams of fat per serving; replace the oil that is called for with one of the fat replacements listed.	Nonfat or light sour cream, applesauce, pineapple juice, or liqueur, depending on the cake.
Homemade cakes and coffee cake	1/4 to 1/3 cup shortening or butter per cake.	Liqueur for some cakes, light sour cream for chocolate ones; fruit juice or purees work well with carrot, apple, and spice cakes.
Cheese sauce	Omit butter; the cheese is the vital fatty ingredient; use a sharp, reduced-fat cheddar.	Make your thickening paste by mixing Wondra flour with a little bit of milk, then whisk in the remaining milk called for in the recipe.
Cookies	Generally you can only cut the fat by half. If the original recipe calls for 1 cup of butter, for example, try cutting it to 1/2 cup.	Fat-free cream cheese for rich cookies; some fruit purees may work in fruit drop cookies. Maple syrup for oatmeal cookies.

Ideal fat thresholds and fat replacements for
different types of recipes

Recipe	Fat Threshold	Fat Replacements
Frosting		Cut the fat in half by using a high-quality diet margarine like I Can't Believe It's Not Butter Light.
Marinades	1 tablespoon canola oil per cup of marinade (or none at all).	Fruit juices or beer to help balance the sharpness of the more acidic ingredients (vinegar, tomato juice).
Muffins and nut breads	2 tablespoons canola oil for a 12-muffin recipe.	Fat-free sour cream, flavored yogurts, fruit purees, maple syrup.
Pie and other pastry crusts	3 tablespoons shortening or canola margarine for every 1 cup flour.	Use fat-free cream cheese and substitute buttermilk for the required water.
Vinaigrette dressings	1 to 2 tablespoons olive or canola oil per 1/2 cup dressing.	Fruit juice, fruit purees (raspberry or pear), light corn syrup, maple syrup, non-alcoholic wines (depending on the recipe).
White sauces and gravies	1 teaspoon butter per serving of sauce.	Add a little more milk or broth to replace the fat. I use whole milk for a rich white sauce because, to me, whole milk *is* cream.

Chapter 5

The 24 Recipes You Cannot Live Without

I hope you will enjoy the collection of recipes in this chapter. There are recipes for everyone in this chapter, including recipes for all types of fiber, so know which fiber sources work best for you. For example, you will find recipes to boost your fiber (such as Raisin Bran muffins) or work whole wheat bread into your day (snickerdoodle toast). There are also recipes that go easy on the intestines (Crock-Pot chicken breasts, salmon in wine sauce, and microwave lemon rice). But mostly you will find low-fat recipes for the high-fat foods we know and love (burgers and fries, spinach manicotti, lasagna, chocolate cream cheese muffins, and more). Don't miss the slow cooker section at the end of this chapter!

Please note: The following is a key to the abbreviations used in the recipes: tablespoon (Tbs.), teaspoon (tsp.), gram (g), milligram (mg), ounces (oz.), and pound (lb.).

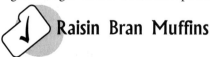 **Raisin Bran Muffins**

This recipe is for people who do well with wheat bran. These muffins are absolutely addictive. They freeze well, so they make a great breakfast on the run or a quick snack or dinner bread.

Makes 18 muffins.

- 1 cup whole wheat flour
- 1 1/2 cups unbleached white flour
- 1 1/4 cups sugar
- 2 1/2 tsp. baking soda
- 1 tsp. salt
- 3 cups Raisin Bran cereal
- 2 cups low-fat buttermilk
- 1/4 cup canola oil
- 1/4 cup maple syrup
- 1 large egg
- 2 egg whites

1. Preheat oven to 425 degrees and line 18 muffin cups with papers (or coat with canola cooking spray).

2. Place flours, sugar, baking soda, and salt in large mixing bowl and beat on low speed of mixer to blend well. Add Raisin Bran and beat on low until blended.

3. Pour buttermilk, oil, maple syrup, and eggs into medium bowl and whisk with fork to blend well. Pour into dry ingredients and beat on low speed briefly, just to blend.

4. Spoon 1/4 cup batter into each prepared muffin cup and bake approximately 15 minutes (until tester inserted in center of muffins comes out clean). Transfer to rack and cool.

Note: You can cover the mixing bowl and chill the muffin batter in the refrigerator for up to one week, although the mixture will thicken.

Per muffin: 197 calories, 4.5 g protein, 37 g carbohydrate, 4 g fat (.5 g saturated fat), 12 mg cholesterol, 3 g fiber, 370 mg sodium. Calories from fat: 18 percent.

Blueberry Oat Bran Streusel Muffins

Makes 12 muffins.

Streusel topping

- 3 Tbs. unbleached flour
- 3 Tbs. sugar
- 1/2 tsp. ground cinnamon
- 2 Tbs. canola margarine

Blueberries

- 1 1/2 cups fresh or frozen blueberries
- 1 to 2 Tbs. flour (optional)

Batter

- 2/3 cup oat bran
- 2/3 cup unbleached flour
- 2/3 cup whole wheat flour
- 2 tsp. baking powder
- 1/2 tsp. salt
- 2 tbs. canola margarine
- 1/3 cup light corn syrup
- 1/3 cup granulated sugar
- 1 egg
- 2 egg whites (or 1/4 cup egg substitute)
- 1 tsp. vanilla extract
- 1/4 tsp. grated lemon peel (lemon zest)
- 1/2 cup milk (low-fat or whole)

1. Preheat oven to 375 degrees. Line 12 muffin cups with papers (or coat with canola cooking spray).

2. Make struesel topping: Place flour, sugar, and cinnamon in small bowl and blend well. Cut in margarine with fork until mixture resembles course crumbs; set aside.

3. Prepare blueberries: In small bowl, sprinkle flour over blueberries if desired (to keep the blueberries from turning the batter purple); set aside.

4. Prepare batter: Combine oat bran, flours, baking powder, and salt in medium bowl.

5. In mixer bowl, beat margarine, corn syrup, and sugar at medium speed until light and fluffy. Add egg and egg whites, beating until smooth. Add vanilla and lemon peel.

6. On lowest speed, beat in dry ingredients, alternating with the milk, just until blended (do not overmix). Fold blueberries into the batter gently.

7. Spoon 1/4 cup of batter into each muffin cup. Sprinkle with streusel topping. Bake approximately 20 minutes or until toothpick inserted in center of muffin comes out clean. Cool in pans on wire rack.

Per serving (made with low-fat milk): 186 calories, 4 g protein, 34 g carbohydrate, 4.9 g fat (.9 g saturated fat), 18 mg cholesterol, 3 g fiber, 233 mg sodium. Calories from fat: 23 percent.

Note: These muffins freeze well; reheat in microwave.

Pumpkin Pecan Wheat Bread

Makes 10 slices.

- 3/4 cup unbleached white flour
- 1/2 cup plus 2 Tbs. whole wheat flour
- 1 1/2 tsp. pumpkin pie spice
- 1 tsp. baking powder
- 1/2 tsp. baking soda
- 1/4 tsp. salt
- 1/4 cup finely chopped pecans
- 3 Tbs. canola margarine or butter, softened
- 1/4 cup plus 1 Tbs. light or fat-free cream cheese

- 1/2 cup granulated sugar
- 1/2 cup packed dark brown sugar
- 1 large egg
- 2 Tbs. egg substitute or 1 egg white
- 1/2 cup solid-pack pumpkin
- 1 tsp. finely chopped orange zest
- 2 Tbs. concentrated orange juice (or orange liqueur)

1. Preheat oven to 350 degrees. Coat an 8 1/2 × 4 1/2 loaf pan with canola cooking spray (or oil) and lightly flour.
2. Combine flours, pumpkin pie spice, baking powder, baking soda, salt, and pecans in medium bowl.
3. In a large bowl, using an electric mixer, cream the margarine or butter and cream cheese. Add the sugars and beat until light.
4. Add the egg and egg substitute or egg white and beat well.
5. Beat in pumpkin, orange zest, and orange juice.
6. Add the dry ingredients to the pumpkin mixture and mix just until blended. Spoon into prepared pan and smooth out top with spatula. Bake for approximately 45 minutes or until toothpick inserted in center comes out clean. Cool for 10 minutes. Remove from pan; cool completely on wire rack.

Per serving: 212 calories, 4.5 g protein, 32.5 g carbohydrate, 7.5 g fat (2 g saturated fat), 26 mg cholesterol, 2 g fiber, 235 mg sodium. Calories from fat: 32 percent.

Snickerdoodle Wheat Toast

If snickerdoodle cookies could be a breakfast bread, this would be it. Whole wheat bread gives this breakfast treat a shot of fiber, and canola margarine keeps it tasting buttery without all the saturated fat.

Makes 5 snickerdoodle toasts.

- 2 Tbs. canola margarine (butter or another margarine can be used)
- 3 tsp. granulated sugar
- 3/4 tsp. ground cinnamon
- 5 slices whole wheat bread (about 40 grams each)

1. Place margarine, sugar, and cinnamon into a custard cup or similar. Blend with a fork or spoon until ingredients are completely mixed and a spread is formed.
2. Toast bread and spread it with the snickerdoodle mixture.

Per snickerdoodle toast: 150 calories, 4 g protein, 21 g carbohydrate, 6 g fat (.8 g saturated fat), 0 mg cholesterol, 2.5 g fiber, 254 mg sodium. Calories from fat: 35 percent.

Wheat Focaccia With Marinara and Cheese

At first glance, it looks like this recipe takes a long time to make, but it actually goes very quickly—and you don't even need a bread machine! Served with soup and vegetables, this pizza-like bread makes a light meal.

Makes 12 servings.

- 2 Tbs. extra-virgin olive oil
- 2 cloves garlic, minced or pressed (omit if you have trouble with garlic)

Dough:

- 1 3/4 cups warm water (110 to 115 degrees)
- 1 Tbs. sugar
- 1 package (1 tablespoon) rapid-rise yeast
- 2 1/2 cups whole wheat flour
- 2 1/2 cups unbleached white flour

- 2 Tbs. extra virgin olive oil
- 1 tsp. salt

Topping and prep:

- Olive or canola cooking spray
- 1/3 cup shredded Parmesan cheese
- 3/4 tsp. dried oregano
- 1/4 to 1/2 tsp. salt
- 2/3 cup bottled marinara sauce
- 4 oz. part-skim mozzarella cheese, grated (1 cup packed)

1. Combine the 2 tablespoons oil and garlic in a small cup and set aside. (If possible, allow the mixture to steep overnight before using.)

2. In medium bowl, combine the water, sugar, and yeast and gently stir until yeast is dissolved. Let stand 5 minutes or until foamy.

3. Stir 1 cup of the flour into the yeast mixture, then stir in the oil and salt. Stir in remaining flour. Knead briefly on a floured surface to incorporate the flour.

4. Let the dough rest approximately 10 minutes while you preheat the oven to 450 degrees and prepare the pan. (Generously coat a 13 × 9 baking pan with cooking spray.)

5. Turn the dough into the pan and pat out evenly with your fingertips. Flour your fingertips and make indentations in the surface of the dough at 1-inch intervals. Spread the reserved garlic-oil mixture evenly over the dough with your fingertips.

6. In a small bowl, stir together the Parmesan cheese, oregano, and salt (or combine in a mini-food processor). Sprinkle the dough with the cheese mixture. Bake for 15 to 20 minutes or until the top is nicely browned. Turn the oven off. Spread the marinara

sauce evenly over the focaccia. Top with mozzarella cheese and put it back in the warm oven until the cheese is melted (approximately 3 minutes). Cut into rectangles and serve warm.

Per serving: 274 calories, 10.3 g protein, 41.3 g carbohydrate, 8 g fat (2.4 g saturated fat), 7 mg cholesterol, 4 g fiber, 413 mg sodium. Calories from fat: 26 percent.

 ## Hero Sandwiches With Reduced-Fat Russian Dressing

Makes 3 sandwiches.

- 6 large slices whole wheat bread (half of a one-pound loaf of unsliced French bread can also be used)
- 3 Tbs. Russian dressing (recipe on next page)
- 2 Tbs. chopped green onion (optional)
- 1/2 cucumber, sliced (optional)
- 6 ounces sliced very lean premium ham
- 4 ounces sliced reduced-fat Swiss or light Jarlsberg cheese
- 1 tomato, sliced

1. With a sharp knife, cut the bread horizontally in half. In a small bowl, mix the Russian dressing with the chopped green onion.

2. On the bottom of 3 slices of bread, layer the cucumber slices, ham, cheese, and tomato.

3. Spread the Russian dressing generously on top. Replace the top of bread. Slice into equal pieces to serve.

Per serving (using whole wheat bread): 454 calories, 31 g protein, 50.5 g carbohydrate, 15.5 g fat (6 g saturated fat), 48 mg cholesterol, 6.3 g fiber, 1,600 mg sodium. Calories from fat: 30 percent.

Russian Dressing

Makes 5 tablespoons.

- 1 Tbs. canola mayonnaise
- 1 Tbs. light or fat-free sour cream
- 2 Tbs. ketchup
- 1/4 tsp. hot sauce or chili sauce
- 1 tsp. sugar
- 1 1/2 tsp. seasoned rice vinegar, white wine vinegar, or white vinegar
- 1 tsp. lemon juice
- 1/4 tsp. Worcestershire sauce
- 1/8 tsp. salt
- a pinch or two of freshly ground pepper

Combine all ingredients in a small bowl; stir well to blend. The dressing can be stored, covered, in the refrigerator for up to two weeks; stir before serving.

Reduced-Fat Burger and Fries

To time your cooking so the burger and fries are done at the same time, preheat the oven for the fries, then mix up the burger mixture and press into patties. Start cooking the fries, then proceed to the burgers.

Makes 4 servings.

Burgers:

- 1 lb. ground sirloin or any extra-lean ground beef
- 2 Tbs. bottled steak sauce
- 1/4 to 1/2 cup finely chopped onion (optional)
- 1/4 cup egg substitute or 1 beaten egg

- freshly ground black pepper
- garlic salt
- canola cooking spray
- 4 whole grain hamburger buns
- optional toppings: 4 thin slices reduced-fat cheese (sharp cheddar or Monterey Jack), ketchup, mustard, lettuce, and sliced tomato.

1. In a large bowl, mix together ground beef, steak sauce, egg substitute, and onion (if desired).

2. Divide mixture into 4 portions and shape into 1/2-inch-thick patties.

3. Lightly sprinkle pepper and garlic salt on both sides of each burger.

4. Spray grill rack or pan with canola cooking spray. Grill the burgers over a medium flame, or pan-fry over medium heat in a nonstick frying pan for about 5 minutes on each side or until they're cooked through.

5. If you like, top burgers with cheese in the final 30 seconds of cooking.

6. Serve the burgers on toasted buns and top as desired.

Fries:

- 12 oz. Ore Ida Country Style French Fries (frozen)

1. Preheat oven to 450 degrees.

2. Arrange frozen fries in a single layer on a thick baking sheet.

3. Bake in center of oven for approximately 15 to 20 minutes or until desired color and crispness.

Per serving (burger and fries): 422 calories, 25 g protein, 43.5 g carbohydrate, 16 g fat (5 g saturated fat), 31 mg cholesterol, 6 g fiber, 697 mg sodium. Calories from fat: 34 percent.

Spinach Ricotta Manicotti With Alfredo Sauce

Makes 4 to 5 dinner entrees.

Light Alfredo Sauce:

- 1 Tbs. butter
- 2 cups whole milk, divided use (fat-free half-and-half can also be used)
- 4 Tbs. Wondra flour
- 1/8 tsp. nutmeg
- 1/8 tsp. white pepper
- 1/4 cup shredded Parmesan cheese

Melt butter in medium saucepan or microwave-safe medium bowl. Stir in 1/4 cup of the milk, flour, nutmeg, and pepper. Slowly stir in remaining milk. Cook on high in microwave (stirring every 2 minutes) or over medium-low heat on the stove (stirring constantly) until sauce thickens slightly. This will take approximately 3 or 4 minutes on the stove or in the microwave. Stir in Parmesan cheese.

Manicotti:

- 10-oz. box frozen, chopped spinach
- 15-oz. container part-skim ricotta cheese
- 3/4 cup freshly grated Parmesan cheese
- 1/2 cup egg substitute
- 4 Tbs. minced fresh parsley leaves (preferably flat leaf)
- salt and pepper to taste
- 8 to 10 manicotti shells cooked according to package directions
- 8 to 10 thin slices prosciutto (approx. 3 oz.)
- 2 cups light alfredo sauce (see previous recipe)

1. Preheat oven to 350 degrees. Coat a 9 × 13 baking pan with canola cooking spray.

2. Place spinach, ricotta, Parmesan, egg substitute, and parsley in mixing bowl and beat on low to blend well. Add salt and pepper to taste.

3. Fill each cooled manicotti shell with approximately 1/3 cup of the filling. Place in the prepared pan and lay a slice of prosciutto over each.

4. Pour Alfredo sauce evenly over manicotti. Bake in middle of oven approximately 30 minutes. Let stand 10 minutes before serving.

Per serving (if 5 servings per recipe): 454 calories, 30.5 g protein, 43.5 g carbohydrate, 17.5 g fat (10 g saturated fat), 55 mg cholesterol, 2.5 g fiber, 642 mg sodium. Calories from fat: 35 percent.

Note: My original recipe contains 620 calories, 36 g fat (21 g saturated fat), and 190 mg cholesterol per serving.

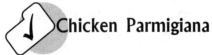

Chicken Parmigiana

Chicken Parmigiana is one of my favorite restaurant entrees. This recipe is much lower in fat and will hopefully work better for you than the restaurant version.

Makes 4 servings.

- 1/2 cup egg substitute
- 3/4 cup Italian-style or plain bread crumbs
- 1/8 tsp. freshly ground pepper
- 4 boneless, skinless chicken breasts, pounded well with a meat mallet to even the thickness
- olive or canola cooking spray
- 2 tsp. olive or canola oil

- 1/3 cup beer, sherry, or white wine (optional)
- 1 1/2 cups bottled marinara sauce
- 3/4 cup grated part-skim mozzarella cheese (or 3 oz. thinly sliced)
- 2 to 3 Tbs. grated Parmesan cheese

1. Put the egg substitute in a pie plate. On waxed paper, blend the bread crumbs with the pepper. Dip the chicken breasts first in the egg, then in the bread crumbs, then repeat to coat well. Set each piece of chicken aside on a plate.

2. Coat a large, heavy nonstick skillet generously with cooking spray. Add the oil and heat over medium-high heat until hot. Add the chicken and brown on the bottom, approximately 5 minutes. Spray the tops of the chicken with cooking spray, flip over, and brown on the second side, approximately 5 minutes. Add the beer if the pan seems dry.

3. When the chicken is brown on both sides, spoon the sauce over each breast, top with the mozzarella, and sprinkle with the Parmesan. Reduce the heat to low, cover and continue cooking for approximately three to five minutes, or until the cheese is melted.

Per serving: 394 calories, 41 g protein, 25 g carbohydrate, 14 g fat (4.7 g saturated fat), 87 mg cholesterol, 1 g fiber, 600–1,000 mg sodium. Calories from fat: 33 percent.

Note: The original recipe (using veal) contains 669 calories, 250 mg cholesterol, and 41 g fat!

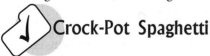

Crock-Pot Spaghetti

This is a family favorite. We make it every single week.

Makes 4 servings.

- canola cooking spray
- 1 lb. ground sirloin or other extra-lean ground beef
- 25-oz. bottle marinara sauce (about 2 3/4 cups)
- 4 garlic cloves, minced or pressed (omit if garlic isn't well tolerated)
- 1 onion, chopped (omit if onion isn't well tolerated)
- 4 to 6 cups cooked whole wheat blend spaghetti noodles

1. Coat a large, nonstick frying pan with canola cooking spray. Set heat to medium. Add ground sirloin, breaking it up into small pieces with spatula. Cook, stirring occasionally, until nicely browned. Place in Crock-Pot.

2. Pour marinara sauce into Crock-Pot. Add garlic and/or onion, as desired. Stir well to blend.

3. Cover, turn Crock-Pot to low, and cook approximately 8 to 10 hours (3 hours on high).

4. Stir spaghetti noodles into Crock-Pot, or spoon each serving of sauce over a serving of cooked noodles.

Per serving: 421 calories, 32.5 g protein, 55 g carbohydrate, 8 g fat (3 g saturated fat), 69 mg cholesterol, 3.5 g fiber, 800 mg sodium. Calories from fat: 17 percent.

Mini Meat Loaf Au Gratin

Many meat loaf recipes can cause problems because they are often high in fat (some contain sausage meat) or spicy or both. This recipe is a mild but flavorful version of this American classic. You can freeze the loaves and pull them out when you need a quick dinner for one or two.

Makes 5 mini loaves.

- 5 aluminum mini loaf pans (3 1/2 × 6), available in most supermarkets
- 2 lb. ground sirloin or other extra-lean ground beef
- 1/4 cup egg substitute
- 3/4 cup reduced-fat sharp cheddar cheese
- 1 small onion, chopped (omit if onion causes you trouble)
- 1/3 cup plain bread crumbs
- 1 1/2 Tbs. Worcestershire sauce
- 1 Tbs. Dijon or prepared mustard
- 1/2 tsp. salt
- 1/2 tsp. pepper
- 1 1/4 cups tomato sauce

1. Preheat oven to 350 degrees. Coat 5 mini loaf pans with canola cooking spray.

2. Add ground beef, egg substitute, cheese, onion, bread crumbs, Worcestershire sauce, mustard, salt, and pepper to large bowl. Mix well with hands or wooden spoon.

3. Add approximately 1 cup of the mixture to each prepared loaf pan. Bake about 25 minutes. Pour approximately 1/4 cup of tomato sauce over each mini loaf while in the pan and bake an additional 5 to 8 minutes to heat tomato sauce.

Serving suggestion: Serve each mini meat loaf with 1/2 cup steamed brown rice and 1/2 cup peas and carrots.

Per serving (just meat loaf): 339 calories, 36 g protein, 12 g carbohydrate, 15.5 g fat (6.8 g saturated fat), 58 mg cholesterol, 2 g fiber, 815 mg sodium. Calories from fat: 43 percent.

Per serving (when served with rice, peas, and carrots): 517 calories, 41 g protein, 50 g carbohydrate, 16 g fat (7 g saturated fat), 58 mg cholesterol, 7 g fiber, 882 mg sodium. Calories from fat: 29 percent.

Quick and Mild (No-Boil) Lasagna

Here is a low-fat, quick, mild recipe for no-boil lasagna. It's a favorite in my house.

Makes 8 servings.

- 3/4 lb. ground sirloin or other extra-lean ground beef
- 26-oz. jar marinara (or spaghetti) sauce with 2 g of fat per serving
- 14 1/2-oz. can vegetable or chicken broth
- 15-oz. container part-skim or low-fat ricotta cheese
- 1 cup grated part-skim mozzarella cheese
- 5 Tbs. grated Parmesan cheese
- 3 Tbs. chopped fresh parsley or 1 tbs. dried parsley
- 3 Tbs. chopped fresh basil leaves (optional)
- 1/4 cup egg substitute
- 1/2 tsp. salt (optional)
- 1/4 tsp. pepper
- 9 wide lasagna noodles—uncooked, about 9.6 oz. (whole wheat blend noodles can also be used if available)

1. Preheat oven to 350 degrees. In large, nonstick saucepan, brown ground sirloin well. Stir in marinara sauce and broth and set aside.

2. In medium bowl, combine ricotta, 3/4 cup of the mozzarella, 3 tablespoons Parmesan cheese, parsley, basil, egg substitute, salt, and pepper.

3. In 13 × 9 baking dish, layer 1 1/2 cups meat sauce and then 3 strips of uncooked noodles. Dot the noodles with 1/3 of the cheese mixture. Cover the cheese with 1 1/2 cups meat sauce and 3 more strips of noodles. Dot the noodles with another 1/3 of the

cheese mixture. Top the cheese with 1 1/2 cups meat sauce and the last 3 noodles. Dot the noodles with the remaining cheese mixture and meat sauce. Sprinkle the remaining 2 tablespoons Parmesan and 1/4 cup mozzarella over the top.

4. Spray one side of foil with canola cooking spray (so the cheese doesn't stick) and cover the lasagna tightly. Bake for 35 minutes. Uncover and bake 15 more minutes. Let stand 10 minutes.

Per serving: 346 calories, 24 g protein, 34.5 g carbohydrate, 12 g fat (6 g saturated fat), 38 mg cholesterol, 3 g fiber, 935 mg sodium. Calories from fat: 31 percent.

Classic Oatmeal-Raisin Cookies

Chocolate can give some people with IBS trouble, and so can high-fat treats. This reduced-fat version of classic oatmeal-raisin cookies, with half the fat and 28 percent fewer calories than the original, is a great, chewy alternative to chocolate chip cookies.

Makes about 32 large cookies.

- 1/4 cup plus 1/8 cup canola margarine or butter, softened (margarine must have 11 grams of fat per tablespoon to work the same as butter in this recipe)
- 1/4 cup plus 1/8 cup fat-free or light cream cheese
- 1 cup packed brown sugar
- 1/2 cup sugar
- 1/4 cup low-fat buttermilk
- 1/4 cup egg substitute
- 2 Tbs. maple syrup
- 2 tsp. vanilla extract
- 1 cup unbleached white flour (whole wheat flour can also be used)

- 1/2 tsp. baking soda
- 1 1/2 tsp. ground cinnamon
- 1/4 tsp. salt
- 3 cups quick or old-fashioned oats
- 1 cup raisins
- 1/2 cup chopped walnuts (optional)

1. Preheat oven to 350 degrees. Coat 2 thick cookie sheets or baking stones with canola cooking spray.

2. In a large bowl, beat the butter with the cream cheese. Beat in the sugars, buttermilk, egg substitute, maple syrup, and vanilla, and beat until light and fluffy.

3. Combine the flour, baking soda, cinnamon, and salt; beat into the butter mixture, mixing well. Stir in the oats, raisins, and nuts, mixing well.

4. Drop spoonfuls of dough 2 inches apart on the prepared cookie sheets.

5. Bake one cookie sheet at a time in the upper third of the oven for approximately 10 minutes, or until lightly browned. Transfer the cookies to wire racks to cool completely. Store in airtight container.

Per cookie: 115 calories, 2.5 g protein, 21 g carbohydrate, 2.7 g fat (.4 g saturated fat), .3 mg cholesterol, 1.2 g fiber, 77 mg sodium. Calories from fat: 21 percent.

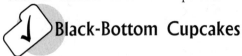

Black-Bottom Cupcakes

This is a reduced-fat version of the popular black-bottom cupcakes/muffins. Although the chocolate and fat are scaled down, these muffins are still totally addictive and delicious. They are great when you need a quick chocolate fix.

Makes 18 cupcakes.

Cream cheese filling:

- 3/4 cup Neufchâtel or light cream cheese, softened (fat-free can also be used)
- 1 tsp. vanilla extract
- 1/3 cup plus 1 tablespoon sugar
- 1 large egg

Muffin batter:

- 3/4 cup unbleached white flour
- 3/4 cup whole wheat flour
- 1 cup sugar
- 1/4 cup unsweetened cocoa
- 1 tsp. baking soda
- 1/2 tsp. salt
- 1 cup water
- 2 Tbs. canola oil
- 3 Tbs. light or fat-free sour cream
- 1 Tbs. white vinegar
- 1 1/2 tsp. vanilla extract
- 1/3 cup chopped almonds (optional)
- 2 Tbs. sugar (optional)

1. Preheat oven to 350 degrees. Line 18 muffin cups with paper cups.

2. Make cream cheese filling by beating the ingredients together in a small bowl until smooth; set aside.

3. In a large bowl, combine the flours, sugar, cocoa, baking soda, and salt; mix well. Add the water, oil, sour cream, vinegar, and vanilla. Using an electric mixer, beat for 2 minutes on medium speed.

4. Fill the muffin cups half full with the batter. Top each with a tablespoon of the cream cheese mixture. Sprinkle chopped almonds and sugar over the top if desired.

5. Bake for 20 minutes, or until the cream cheese mixture is light golden brown. Cool for 15 minutes; remove from the pans. Cool completely. Store in the refrigerator.

Per serving: 143 calories, 3 g protein, 25 g carbohydrate, 3.7 g fat (1.5 g saturated fat), 17 mg cholesterol, 2 g fiber, 185 mg sodium. Calories from fat: 23 percent.

 ## Microwave Lemon Rice

Makes 4 servings.

- 1 1/2 cups unrinsed basmati rice (brown rice can also be used)
- 2 1/4 cups chicken broth
- 2 to 3 Tbs. lemon juice
- 2/3 cup frozen petite green peas (if tolerated)
- salt and pepper to taste

1. Place rice, broth, and lemon juice in 2- or 3-quart microwave-safe dish. Cook on high, uncovered, approximately 15 to 17 minutes, or until steam holes appear in rice.
2. Sprinkle peas over rice, cover dish, and cook on high approximately 5 to 7 minutes or until rice is fully cooked and peas are lightly cooked.
3. Fluff with fork and serve.

Per serving: 296 calories, 9 g protein, 60 g carbohydrate, 1.3 g fat (.4 g saturated fat), 0 mg cholesterol, 2 g fiber, 460 mg sodium. Calories from fat: 4 percent.

Microwave Orange Tapioca Pudding

If you don't care for orange, then try lemon curd or apple butter with the tapioca instead.

Makes 6 servings.

- 1/4 cup sugar (you can use less if desired)
- 3 Tbs. Minute tapioca
- 2 3/4 cups low-fat milk
- 1/4 cup egg substitute
- 2 Tbs. orange marmalade (lemon curd or apple butter can be substituted)
- 1 tsp. vanilla

1. Mix sugar, tapioca, milk, egg, and marmalade in microwavable bowl. Microwave on high 10 to 12 minutes until mixture comes to a full boil, stirring every 2 minutes.

2. Stir in vanilla. Cool 20 minutes; stir. Spoon into serving dishes. Serve warm or chilled. Store in refrigerator.

Per serving: 127 calories, 5 g protein, 22.5 g carbohydrate, 2 g fat (1.3 g saturated fat), 8 mg cholesterol, 0 g fiber, 73 mg sodium. Calories from fat: 14 percent.

 ## Turkey Teriyaki Burger

Makes 6 burgers.

- 1 lb. ground turkey
- 1 cup steamed rice (leftover rice works fine)
- 1/2 tsp. chopped or minced ginger (omit if you don't tolerate ginger well)
- 1/4 cup teriyaki sauce
- canola cooking spray
- 6 sesame seed whole grain buns
- optional toppings: soy sauce or sweet and sour sauce, lettuce, and tomato slices

1. Place turkey, rice, ginger, and teriyaki sauce to large bowl; blend well using a spoon or your hands.

2. Divide mixture evenly into 6 portions. Form into 1/2-inch thick burgers.

3. Spray grill rack or nonstick skillet with cooking spray. Grill or pan-fry over medium heat. Cook about 4 minutes on each side, or until nicely browned and cooked through. Serve each burger on a toasted bun with desired toppings.

Per serving: 279 calories, 16 g protein, 34 g carbohydrate, 8.3 g fat (2.5 g saturated), 46 mg cholesterol, 5 g fiber, 780 mg sodium. Calories from fat: 27 percent.

 ## Microwaved Salmon in Wine Sauce

Makes 2 or 3 servings.
- 1 1/2 tsp. olive oil
- 2 6-oz. or 3 4-oz. center-cut salmon fillets (about 1 1/2-inches thick at thickest part, skin and bones removed)
- 2 Tbs. dry white wine
- 1 Tbs. finely chopped fresh parsley
- 1 tsp. fresh, dried, or frozen chives (optional)
- garlic salt to taste
- freshly ground black pepper to taste

Suggested side dishes:
- 3 cups steamed brown rice or cooked whole wheat blend noodles
- 3 cups steamed vegetables of your choice

1. Coat a square, microwave-safe casserole dish with canola cooking spray. Place the salmon pieces in dish, folding the thin sides under if necessary so the fillets

are of even thickness. Drizzle the wine and olive oil over the salmon and sprinkle parsley, chives, garlic salt, and pepper over the top. Cover the casserole (or use microwave-safe plastic wrap to cover dish).

2. Microwave on high for 6 minutes. If your microwave does not have a turntable, turn the casserole a quarter turn every 2 minutes so the fish cooks evenly. Take the casserole dish out, and let it stand a few minutes (without uncovering).

3. Test the salmon in the thickest part with a fork. If it isn't cooked throughout, heat another minute or two until done. Serve each salmon fillet on a mound of rice and spoon the wine sauce (the sauce in the bottom of the dish) over the top.

Per serving (including brown rice and a green vegetable) if 3 servings per recipe: 498 calories, 33 g protein, 66 g carbohydrate, 10.5 g fat (1.4 g saturated fat), 62 mg cholesterol, 7 g fiber, 100 mg sodium. Calories from fat: 19 percent.

Get Crocked (with your slow cooker!)

Dr. Frissora recommends the slow cooker to her patients with IBS and believe it or not, the slow cooker is actually one of my favorite appliances. I like that I can leave it "on" while I'm out of the house and if I'm an hour late getting home, it's no big deal. There is a wonderful sense of comfort knowing your dinner is cooking at home while you are away. If you need to keep things warm for another hour, because your family or dinner guests are delayed, just keep the slow cooker on low for another hour. It's just that simple!

Cooking vegetables and meats the "slow but sure" way (with a minimum of fat) can work wonders with an irritable bowel. Here are just a few of my favorite slow-cooker recipes to get you started.

Country Pot Roast

This recipe includes directions with or without a slow cooker.
Makes at least 6 servings.

- 3- to 5-lb. center-cut cross-rib (shoulder) roast, trimmed of visible fat
- 1/4 cup unbleached white flour
- 1 1/2 tsp. canola oil
- 1 cup tomato juice, tomato sauce, or bottled marinara sauce
- 3 garlic cloves, minced (omit if you have a problem with garlic)
- 4 carrots, sliced
- 3 large potatoes, quartered
- 1 large onion, coarsely chopped (omit if you have a problem with onion)
- 1 cup sliced celery
- 1 tsp. salt
- 1 1/2 tsp. dried oregano
- 1/4 tsp. freshly ground pepper

1. Place the roast on a cutting board or waxed paper and coat with the flour.
2. Heat the oil in a Dutch oven or large saucepan over medium-high heat. Add the roast and cook until browned on all sides.
3. If using a slow cooker, add roast to cooker along with all remaining ingredients. Set to high and cook for 3 to 4 hours (depending on the size of the roast), or on low for 7 to 8 hours. Proceed to Step 4. If not using a slow cooker, add all the remaining ingredients and bring to a boil. Reduce heat to low, cover pot, and simmer for 2 to 4 hours, depending on the size of

the roast, or until the meat is fork-tender, turning several times.

4. Transfer meat to a cutting board. In batches, puree the cooking liquid and vegetables in a blender at high speed. Pour back into the pan or into a serving bowl. Slice the roast and serve with the vegetable gravy.

Per serving: 405 calories, 37 g protein, 39.5 g carbohydrate, 13 g fat (5 g saturated fat), 90 mg cholesterol, 5 g fiber, 606 mg sodium. Calories from fat: 29 percent.

Note: Standard pot roast recipes contain more than 600 calories and 38 grams of fat per serving!

Orange Cranberry Chicken

This recipe goes great with steamed brown rice.

Makes 6 servings.

- 1 Tbs. low-fat margarine
- 1/3 cup less sugar orange marmalade
- 1/2 cup dried cranberries
- 1/4 cup brown sugar, packed
- 1 tablespoon rice vinegar
- 1 teaspoon chopped ginger
- 1/2 teaspoon ground cinnamon
- 1 cup low-sodium chicken broth (if using broth powder, make it double strength by adding 1 cup of hot water to 2 teaspoons of broth powder)
- 6 skinless, boneless chicken breasts (cut into about 3 pieces each)

1. Add all of the ingredients (except chicken) to the slow cooker and stir well with spoon.

2. Add the chicken to the slow cooker, cover, and cook on high for 3 hours or on low for about 6 hours, until chicken is cooked throughout.

3. Serve chicken with orange cranberry sauce.

Per serving: 253 calories, 28 g protein, 25 g carbohydrate, 4.4 g fat, 1.1 g saturated fat, 73 mg cholesterol, 1 g fiber, 210 mg sodium. Calories from fat: 16 percent.

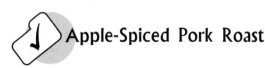

Apple-Spiced Pork Roast

This dish works well with steamed yams or sweet potatoes. Any leftover sliced pork works well for sandwiches the next day too.

Makes 6 servings.

- 2 tsp. finely chopped fresh rosemary
- 2 tsp. finely chopped fresh thyme
- 1 tsp. dried marjoram (dried sage can be substituted)
- 1/2 tsp. salt
- 1/2 tsp. white or black pepper
- 2 1/3 to 2 1/2 pounds pork sirloin tri-tip roast
- 1 cup spiced apple cider (bottled)
- 2 fuji or Granny Smith apples, cored and cut into 3/4-inch pieces
- 1 large red onion, cut into 3/4-inch pieces
- 1/4 cup dark brown sugar, loosely packed
- 1/2 tsp. ground cinnamon
- 2 Tbs. maple butter (maple syrup can be used)
- 2 Tbs. Wondra quick-mixing flour

1. In a small bowl, mix together rosemary, thyme, marjoram, salt, and pepper. Rub the herb mixture all over the outside of the pork roast. Place in the slow cooker. Pour apple cider around the roast. Cover roast with apple pieces, then top apples with onion pieces. Sprinkle brown sugar and cinnamon over the top of the apples and onions.

2. Cover and cook on low for 4 to 5 hours (meat thermometer inserted into the center of roast should register at 165 degrees). When cooked throughout, remove pork roast to serving platter.

3. Turn slower cooker to high. Add maple butter to a microwave-safe custard cup and microwave on high for about 5 seconds to soften. Stir in Wondra flour (add a tablespoon of juice from slow cooler if needed). Stir maple paste into the apple-onion-cider mixture in slow cooker. Cook for 30 minutes longer or until thickened nicely. Meanwhile, after pork has cooled slightly (about 10 minutes), cover with foil to keep warm.

4. Serve sliced pork roast with apple onion sauce and steamed yams if desired!

Per serving: 365 calories, 26 g protein, 27 g carbohydrate, 12 g fat, 4 g saturated fat, 107 mg cholesterol, 2 g fiber, 250 mg sodium. Calories from fat: 30 percent.

Slow-Cooker Shepherd's Pie

Makes 4 servings.

- 6 cups cooked, peeled, hot, drained potato quarters (if potatoes are large, cut them into 6 or 8 pieces)
- 2 Tbs. whipped butter or low-fat margarine
- 6 Tbs. fat-free half-and-half (or low-fat milk)
- salt and pepper to taste
- 2 cups cooked lean meat of choice, cut into bite-size pieces (roasted turkey, roast beef, and so on)
- 2 1/4 cups frozen mixed vegetables, lightly cooked or thawed (such as a blend of green beans, wax beans, and baby carrots)
- 10.5-ounce can condensed cream of celery soup (with around 4.5 grams fat per 1/2 cup serving)

- 1/3 cup fat-free sour cream
- 4 green onions, white and part green, chopped
- 3/4 cup shredded reduced-fat sharp cheddar cheese (optional)

1. Add hot potatoes (from colander) directly into large mixing bowl and add the whipped butter and fat-free half-and-half and beat on low until desired texture is achieved.

2. Add salt and pepper to taste. Coat the inside of the slow cooker with canola cooking spray and spread mashed potatoes in the bottom. Sprinkle black pepper over the top if desired. Spread pieces of meat evenly over mashed potatoes. Top with mixed vegetables.

3. Add condensed cream of celery soup to 2-cup measure and stir in sour cream and green onions. Spread mixture over the top of the vegetables in the slow cooker. Sprinkle with black pepper if desired. Cover and cook on high for 2 hours or low for 4 hours. If you are adding the cheese, sprinkle cheese over the top and cook on high until melted (about 20 to 30 minutes more.)

Per serving: 367 calories, 29 g protein, 46 g carbohydrate, 6.8 g fat, 1.1 g saturated fat, 61 mg cholesterol, 6 g fiber, 487 mg sodium. Calories from fat: 17 percent.

Crock-Pot Chicken Breasts

Makes 6 servings.

- 6 boneless, skinless chicken breasts (6 boneless, center-cut pork loin chops, trimmed of fat, can also be used)
- 1/2 cup flour

- 1 1/2 tsp. garlic salt
- 1 tsp. dry mustard
- 1 Tbs. canola oil
- 6 carrots, cut into ¼-inch slices
- 10 3/4-oz. can Campbell's Healthy Request Chicken and Rice Soup
- about 4 1/2 cups brown steamed rice

1. Spray bottom of Crock-Pot with canola cooking spray.
2. Mix flour, garlic salt, and dry mustard in medium-sized bowl. Dredge chicken (or pork chops) in flour mixture.
3. Add oil to large nonstick frying pan or skillet. Over medium heat, brown chicken breasts (or chops) on both sides. Place in Crock-Pot. Cover meat with sliced carrots. Add soup.
4. Cover and cook on low 8 hours.
5. Serve each chicken breast (or chop) over a mound of steamed rice. With slotted spoon, scoop out carrots and serve next to meat. Drizzle gravy over chicken (or chops).

Per serving: 444 calories, 35 g protein, 61.5 g carbohydrate, 5 g fat (1 g saturated fat), 71 mg cholesterol, 5 g fiber, 706 mg sodium. Calories from fat: 11 percent.

Chapter 6

Navigating the Supermarket

Every time you set foot in a supermarket, you are hit with hundreds of advertising claims: "Fat Free," "No Cholesterol," "Multigrain," "Baked, Not Fried." They are designed to entice you. Remember: All these companies are trying to sell you something. They all want a piece of the food dollar pie. So don't be fooled—find out for yourself and *read the nutrition label.*

Some breads boast that they are "multigrain" or "seven grain," but their nutrition labels show they have only one little gram of fiber per serving. Some "wheat" or "multigrain" crackers don't even have one gram of fiber per serving.

Generally, the more you know about a food product, the better off you'll be. What should you be looking for on the label? Start with the portion size. Remember, what the manufacturer thinks is a portion and what you think is a portion could be two very different things. Some products within the same category may even have different serving sizes. For example, some bread labels give the nutrition information for one slice, others for two slices. Some canned baked beans and chili give the nutrition information for a half cup, others one cup. A serving of cereal can be anything from 1/2 cup to 1 1/4 cups.

Once you've mastered that, it's a good idea to get a quick sense of the product's:

- calories.
- fat grams.
- saturated fat grams.
- fiber grams.

That's what the rest of this chapter is here to help you with. We'll be taking a virtual tour of the typical supermarket, noting the calories, fat grams, fiber content, and more for different foods in order to help you master the 10 Food Steps to Freedom. We'll be examining the fiber contents of breads and cereals. We'll be looking at the better-tasting reduced-fat products available in every aisle of the supermarket. So, are you ready? Here we go.

Looking for fiber in all the right places

Does it really matter which breads or cereals contain the most fiber? You bet it does. Think about it. Most people have a sandwich and a bowl of cereal almost every day. If the bread you make your sandwich with contains seven grams of fiber instead of two, and the bowl of cereal you eat has eight grams of fiber instead of two, it can really make a difference day after day. We are talking about getting 15 grams of fiber—instead of four—with just those two foods. We'll start with the breads and cereals with the most fiber and go from there.

Whole wheat breads and bagels

Many breads that seem like they would have tons of fiber, such as multigrain ones, don't. The bottom line is that you have to check the labels of the breads you like to see just how much fiber they really have. The tricky part is that there are a few breads that list the grams of fiber per two slices, and the rest list it per one slice.

	Fiber(g)	Calories	Fat(g)
Breads (per slice)			
EarthGrains:			
Country Hearth 100% Whole Wheat	3	110	1.5
Iron Kids	2	80	1
Mrs. Wright's:			
100% Whole Wheat	2	70	1
Wheat Bread	2	70	1
Winner's Special Recipe Bread	2	70	1
Northwest Grain Country:			
100% Whole Wheat	3	100	1.5
Early American	2	110	1
Oregon Bread:			
Whole Wheat Hazelnut	3	140	4.5
Western Hazelnut	2	130	4.5
Oroweat:			
Light 100% Whole Wheat	3.5	40	0.25
Light Country Potato Bread	3	40	0.25
Light Country Oat Bread	2.5	40	0.5
Light 9-Grain	2.5	40	0.25
100% Whole Wheat	2	90	1
Health Nut	2	100	2
Branola	2	90	1
Honey Wheat Berry	2	90	1
Best Winter Wheat	2	90	3
Roman Meal:			
Sun Grain Bread	2	100	2
Dakota Wheat Bread	2	90	1
Wonder:			
Light Wheat	2.5	40	0.25
Bagels (per bagel)			
Oroweat:			
100% Whole Wheat	9	240	1.5
Health Nut	5	270	4.5
Oat Nut	4	270	4
Multi Grain	4	260	1.5
Sara Lee:			
Honey Wheat	4	250	1

High-fiber cereals

If you eat a breakfast cereal a few times a week, you sit down to about 156 bowls of cereal a year. So whether you choose a whole grain cereal can make a big difference in the amount of fiber you are eating. I'll tell you a secret: What really distinguishes one cereal from another is not its fat and sodium content, it's the sugar and fiber.

The cereals that have a lot more sugar are usually the ones that have a lot less fiber too. The table below lists most of the cereals that have five grams of fiber or more per serving. Notice that Cheerios and Whole Grain Wheaties didn't make the cut.

	Fiber (g)	Fat (g)	Calories
All-Bran Extra Fiber, 1/2 cup	13	1	50
Fiber One, 1/2 cup	13	1	60
All-Bran Original, 1/2 cup	10	1	80
100% Bran, 1/3 cup	8	0.5	80
Kellogg's Raisin Bran, 1 cup	8	1.5	200
Post Raisin Bran, 1 cup	8	1	190
Shredded Wheat 'n Bran, 1 1/4 cups	8	1	200
Bite Size Frosted Mini-Wheats, 1 cup	6	1	200
Cracklin Oat Bran, 3/4 cup	6	7	190
Raisin Bran Crunch, 1 1/4 cups	5	1	210
Total Raisin Bran, 1 cup	5	1	180
Bran Flakes, 3/4 cup	5	0.5	100
Complete Wheat Bran Flakes, 3/4 cup	5	0.5	90
Crunchy Corn Bran, 3/4 cup	5	1	90
Spoon Size Shredded Wheat, 1 cup	5	0.5	170
Mini-Wheats (Raisin), 3/4 cup	5	1	180
Frosted Shredded Wheat, 1 cup	5	1	190
100% Whole Grain Wheat Chex, 1 cup	5	1.5	180
Fruit & Fibre (Dates, Raisins, and Walnuts), 1 cup	5	3	210
Grape Nuts, 1/2 cup	5	1	210
Raisin Nut Bran, 3/4 cup	5	4	200

Beans: A little goes a long way

Some of you might think there is no way you can handle a serving of beans. Maybe you noticed some IBS symptoms after a big bowl of chili. But was it the beans in the chili, the fatty meat in the chili, or the spices? Or was it the fact that you had a big *bowl* of chili instead of a petite cup?

Beans are a quick way to boost your fiber, with half a cup contributing around six grams of fiber. What's more, beans contain both types of fiber, soluble and insoluble. Try a small serving of beans, preferably not in a very fatty or spicy dish, so you can see how you do with that. A bean burrito, either take-out or home-made, might be a good first bet (try low-fat pintos or refried beans with a flour tortilla, a sprinkling of cheese, and mild sauce).

Here are some of the canned bean products I found in my supermarket:

	Fiber (g)	Cal.	Fat(g)	Sod.(mg)
Taco Bell Vegetarian Refried Beans	8	140	2.5	500
Ortega Refried Beans	9	130	2.5	570
Ortega Fat-Free Refried Beans	9	120	0	570
Rosarita Lowfat Black Beans				
Refried Beans	5	90	0.5	460
Rosarita Vegetarian				
Refried Beans	6	100	2	500
B&M Original Baked Beans	6	170	2	380
S&W Chili Beans Zesty Sauce	6	110	1	580
S&W Santa Fe Beans	6	90	0.5	680

See what I mean about the fiber? Pretty impressive, don't you think?

Whole wheat tortillas

Most of you are going to take one look at a package of whole wheat tortillas and go running as fast as you can toward the traditional white flour tortillas. You have to like whole wheat and be very motivated to eat fiber to want them. I personally don't mind them if the filling is particularly flavorful, and with just one torti-lla you can get a whopping nine grams of fiber.

Frozen entrees: Some high-fiber surprises

	Cal.	Fat (%*) (g)	Fib. (g)	Sat. fat(g)	Sod. (mg)
Frozen Pizza					
Wolfgang Puck's Mushroom & Spinach Pizza, half	270	8 (27%)	5	3	380
Wolfgang Puck's Four Cheese Pizza, 1/2 of a 9.25 ounce pizza	360	15 (37%)	5	6	530
Healthy Choice					
Chicken Enchiladas Suiza	280	6 (19%)	5	3	440
Shrimp & Vegetables	270	6 (20%)	6	3	580
Herb Baked Fish	340	7 (19%)	5	1.5	480
Traditional Breast of Turkey	290	4.5 (14%)	5	2	460
Chicken Enchilada Suprema	300	7 (21%)	4	3	560
Lean Cuisine					
Chicken in Peanut Sauce	290	6 (19%)	4	1.5	590
Baked Fish w/ Cheddar Shells	270	6 (20%)	4	2	540
Fiesta Chicken	270	5 (17%)	4	0.5	590
3-Bean Chili	250	6 (22%)	9	2	590
Marie Calender's					
Chili & Cornbread	540	21 (35%)	7	9	2110
Sweet & Sour Chicken	570	15 (24%)	7	2.5	700
Beef Tips in Mushroom Sc.	430	17 (36%)	6	7	1620
Turkey w/ gravy and dressing	500	19 (34%)	4	9	2040
Spaghetti and Meat Sauce	670	25 (34%)	9	11	1160
Stuffed Pasta Trio	640	18 (25%)	5	9	950
Swanson					
Mexican Style Combination	470	18 (34%)	5	6	1610
Chicken Parmigiana	370	17 (41%)	4	5	1010
Turkey Dinner	310	8.5 (25%)	5	2	890

*Percentage of calories from fat

Frozen entrees can come in handy in many situations, whether as a quick lunch during the workweek or as an easy dinner if you live alone or with one other person. The problem with frozen entrees is that the ones that are lower in fat are almost always too low in calories, carbohydrates, and vegetables. So in order to make the entrees more nutritious and satisfying, consider adding fruits and vegetables. You might also need to add some cooked brown rice, whole grain blend noodles, or even grated cheese.

I've listed on page 134 the nutrition information for some of the lower-fat frozen entrees that offer four grams of fiber or more. If you need to watch your sodium intake, keep an eye on the nutrition label, because some frozen entrees have lots of it.

Losing some of the fat in our favorite foods

I left a couple of brands off the tables in this chapter because they flunked my taste test. If my tasters thought they looked or tasted bad, I left them out. I also don't believe in certain fat-free foods, such as cheese, mayonnaise, margarine, or ice cream. However, there is a brand of fat-free sour cream available that actually beat out the light sour creams in our taste test (Naturally Yours brand). Go figure! And as for fat-free cookies and cake, a few rated an "all right," like the fat-free fig bars and angel food cake, but in general, I much prefer a reduced-fat cookie or cake.

Fat-free but full of calories

When you start reducing fat in favorite foods, the tricky part is making sure you don't eat more of them than you normally would. Fat-free doesn't mean calorie-free, and fat-free doesn't mean you can eat the whole box in one sitting. In fact, many of these fat-free products have just as many calories as the full-fat versions. How can that be? In a word: sugar. Sugar, whether it comes from honey, corn syrup, brown sugar, or high fructose corn syrup, can add moisture and help tenderize bakery products. When added to foods such as ice cream, it adds flavor and structure. So I'm not surprised that manufacturers have turned to sugar for assistance while developing reduced-fat and fat-free products. Keep in mind that the majority of the fat-free and lower-fat products on supermarket shelves usually have the same number of calories as the full-fat counterparts (saving us, at most, only 20 calories per serving).

Fat-free can mean satisfaction-free

If these products aren't as satisfying, we're probably more likely to keep on eating and eating in the hope of reaching some level of satisfaction—after all, it's fat-free! So what's a fat-gram and calorie-watching girl to do? *Only select "light" and fat-free products that you truly like* and that satisfy you enough for you to eat modest amounts. Otherwise, don't bother.

For example, I really love Cracker Barrel Light Sharp Cheddar. It is real cheese to me. My family enjoys Louis Rich turkey bacon, and we don't miss real bacon. Reduced Fat Bisquick is a staple in my house. We all think Louis Rich Turkey Franks and Ball Park Lite franks taste terrific. These are the types of products you want to keep buying—the ones that you truly enjoy. Some companies have definitely gone too far.

In my opinion, certain foods simply aren't meant to be fat-free. If you take all the fat out of a food that was mostly fat to begin with, such as mayonnaise, cheese, ice cream, or butter, then what have you really got? Something other than mayonnaise, cheese, ice cream, or butter—that's for sure. It's not fat-free butter, it's just a new kind of yellow goop.

A number of fat-free, sugar-free, or "light" products have successfully hit their optimal level of fat. These are the foods that withstood a modest reduction in fat without a huge loss in taste satisfaction. You'll find them listed in the tables.

Reduced-fat meat products

I love bacon. I'll admit it. But I am quite satisfied with Louis Rich turkey bacon. I make TLT sandwiches (turkey bacon, lettuce, and tomato) for my family every now and then. We tend to also throw Louis Rich Turkey Franks or Ball Park Lite franks on the grill from time to time. The "meatless" Boca breakfast links also contain two grams of fiber per serving. It is the best-tasting meatless breakfast link I have had. (Then again, I had to literally spit out the others.)

	Cal.	Fat (g) (sat. fat)	Chol.(mg)	Sod.(mg)
Bacon (per ounce)				
Louis Rich Turkey Bacon, 2 slices	70	5(2)	30	360
Campfire Canadian Style, 2 slices	25	0.75(.25)	10	375
Hot dogs (per frank)				
Louis Rich	80	6(2)	40	510
Ball Park Lite	100	7(2.5)	25	540
Ball Park Fat-Free Smoked White Turkey franks	40	0(0)	15	530
Hebrew National Reduced-Fat franks	120	10(4.5)	25	360
Salami/pepperoni (per ounce)				
Gallo Light Salami	60	4(1.5)	25	520
Hormel Turkey Pepperoni	80	4(1.5)	40	550
Sausage (per 2 ounces)				
Boca:				
Breakfast Links, 2	80	3(0)	0	350
Healthy Choice:				
Lowfat Smoked Sausage	80	2.5(1)	25	480
Lowfat Polska Kielbasa	80	2.5(1)	25	480
Hillshire Farm:				
Turkey Polska Kielbasa	90	5(2.5)	30	560
Jimmy Dean:				
50% less fat, 2.5 ounces	170	13(4.5)	50	450
Louis Rich:				
Turkey Smoked Sausage	90	6(1.5)	35	850
Turkey Polska Kielbasa	90	6(1.5)	35	850
The Turkey Store:				
Mild turkey breakfast Sausage links	140	11(3)	45	360

Reduced-fat dairy products

Fat-free half-and-half? I tried out this product in my coffee and in a quiche I was making. What's in it, you ask? Basically they make it by taking nonfat milk and a tiny bit of whole milk, sweetening it with a little corn syrup, and pumping in thickener (carrageenan, a fiber from plants that mixes well with water).

When you see fat-free sour cream, you probably think, "why bother?" But there is a brand of fat-free sour cream that actually beat out the reduced-fat (or "light") sour creams in taste. It makes a nice ranch dip, and I use it as a fat replacement in brownie, cake, and muffin recipes. Heck, I even top my baked potato with it. It's from the Naturally Yours brand, and you'll know it by the container's black and white cowhide pattern.

	Cal.	Fat.(g)	Sat. Fat(g)
Cream (per 2 tablespoons)			
Land O'Lakes Fat Free Half-and-Half	20	0	0
Carnation Coffee-Mate Fat Free	20	0	0
Carnation Coffee-Mate Fat Free French Vanilla	50	0	0
International Delight Nondairy Creamer French Vanilla	60	0	0
Sour Cream (per 2 tablespoons)			
Naturally Yours Fat Free Sour Cream	20	0	0
Knudsen Light	40	2.5	1.5

Frozen desserts

I didn't list sugar-free ice creams in the table on page 139 because they usually contain artificial sweeteners, which can encourage intestinal problems for some people. I also bypassed all the fat-free ice creams (unless they were sorbets, which are naturally fat-free) because, frankly, they didn't score well on taste.

	Cal.	Fat (g) (sat. fat)	Sugar (g)	Chol. (mg)
Starbucks Bars (per bar)				
Frappuccino	120	2(1)	18	10
Ben & Jerry's Lowfat Frozen Yogurt (per 1/2 cup)				
Cherry Garcia	170	3(2)	27	20
Chocolate Fudge Brownie	190	2.5(1)	5	30
S'mores	190	2(1)	15	26
Dreyer's Grand Light Ice Cream (per 1/2 cup)				
Peanut Butter Cup	130	5(2.5)	13	20
Vanilla	100	3(2)	11	20
Mint Chocolate Chip	120	4(3)	13	20
Chocolate Fudge Mousse	110	3(2)	13	20
Cookies 'n Cream	120	4(2)	12	20
Cookie Dough	130	5(2.5)	13	20
Coffee Mousse Crunch	120	4(2.5)	13	20
Sorbet (per 1/2 cup)				
Ben & Jerry's				
Purple Passion Fruit fat free	120	0(0)	30	0
Haagen-Dazs Raspberry	120	0(0)	26	0
Haagen-Dazs Zesty Lemon	120	0(0)	28	0
Sherbet (per 1/2 cup)				
Dreyer's Tropical Rainbow	130	1(0.5)	24	5

Reduced-fat cheeses

I love cheese. Cheese is my middle name. Because I've never liked milk as a beverage, I probably have gotten most of the calcium in my bones from cheese. I am very pleased to announce there are some wonderful reduced-fat cheeses out there. Some are harder to find than others, such as my personal favorite, Cracker Barrel Light Sharp Cheddar. I've tasted most of the cheeses in the list on page 140 and have been very pleased with them, whether they were filling my lasagna or topping my tortilla.

	Cal.	Fat (g)	Saturated Fat (g)
Reduced-fat cheese (per oz. unless otherwise noted)			
Precious Low Moisture Part Skim Mozzarella	80	5	3
Kraft 2% Milk Reduced Fat Singles (per 2/3 ounce slice)	45	3	2
Kraft 2% Milk Reduced Fat Sharp Cheddar	90	6	4
Kraft 2% Milk Reduced Fat Monterey Jack	80	6	4
Sargento Light 4 Cheese Mexican (1/4 cup)	70	4.5	3
Sargento Deli Style Swiss	80	4	2.5
Reduced-fat cream cheese (per ounce)			
Philadelphia Fat Free	30	0	0
Ricotta cheese (per 1/4 cup)			
Precious Part Skim	100	6	4

Pasta sauces

I have listed some store-bought sauces that are great low-fat alternatives on page 141. In order to qualify, they had to contain canola or olive oil (the preferred high monounsaturated fat oils). The tomato-based sauces will also contribute those helpful phytochemicals found in cooked tomato products. You can always add extra-lean ground beef, mushrooms, garlic, onion, and spices if you want to dress them up a little.

	Cal.	Fat (g) (sat. fat)	Fib. (g)	Sod. (mg)
Five Brothers:				
Grilled Eggplant and Parmesan	100	3 (0.5)	3	540
Grilled Summer Vegetable	80	3 (0)	3	550
Mushroom and Garlic Grill	90	3 (0)	3	550
Marinara with Burgundy Wine	90	3 (0)	3	480
Classico:				
Tomato and Basil	50	1 (0)	2	390
Fire-Roasted Tomato and Garlic	60	1 (0)	2	390
Sutter Home:				
Italian Style (with fresh onions and herbs)	80	2 (0)	4	520
Barilla:				
Green and Black Olive	80	2.5 (.5)	3	1,010
Roasted Garlic and Onion	80	3.5 (0)	<1	460
Mushroom and Garlic	70	2 (.5)	3	610
Tomato and Basil	70	1.5 (.5)	3	640
Marinara	70	2 (.5)	2	430

Low-fat yogurt

There are scores of brands and flavors of yogurt in the supermarket. Look for brands that contain active yogurt cultures; the bacteria may help some IBS sufferers. Some brands contain artificial sweeteners, cutting the calories and sugar almost in half. These are fine if you aren't sensitive to the artificial sweetener aftertaste.

Canned fruit

Some people with IBS have noticed that they tend to tolerate well-ripened or canned fruit the best. Obviously, well-ripened fruit isn't available year-round, but canned fruit is. Because there are so many choices of fruits canned in juice or light syrup, I thought I'd better list them for you. You can find them on page 142.

	Calories	Fiber (g)
Del Monte:		
Almond Flavored Apricot Halves in light syrup	90	1
Lite Apricot Halves	60	1
Lite Chunky Mixed Fruit	60	1
Cinnamon Flavored Pear Halves	80	1
Raspberry Flavored Sliced Peaches	80	<1
Dole:		
Pineapple Chunks in their own juice	60	1
Geisha:		
Mandarin Orange in light syrup	70	1
S&W:		
Sun Apricots (almond flavored) in light syrup	90	1
Sun Peaches Tropical in light syrup	80	0
Sweet Memory Peaches in light syrup	80	<1
Natural Style Fruit Cocktail in lightly sweetened fruit juice	80	2
Natural Style Sliced Bartlett Pears	80	2
Natural Style Sliced Cling Peaches	80	1

Psyllium and similar fiber supplement products

Psyllium is a naturally grown and harvested grain that is very good at absorbing and holding moisture. In your intestines, the psyllium swells, theoretically forming an easily eliminated stool. Some people swear by psyllium supplements; others say they have little effect.

The Food and Drug Administration recently recognized that diets containing soluble fiber from psyllium husk may reduce the risk of heart disease by lowering cholesterol when included as part of a low-fat diet. You can find psyllium in the medical aisle of your supermarket. In the pharmacy, they'll be with all the other gastrointestinal products. But finding them is the easy part—once you do you'll wonder:

- Which brand do I buy?
- Do I want flavored and artificially sweetened or unflavored?
- If flavored, do I want to try orange or mint?
- Do I want smooth or regular texture?

And you thought it would be simple. Here is some information that might help you in your quest for psyllium.

Warning

Many of the products warn, "Taking this product without adequate fluid may cause it to swell and block your throat or esophagus and may cause choking. Do not take this product if you have difficulty in swallowing. If you experience chest pain, vomiting, or difficulty in swallowing or breathing after taking this product, seek immediate medical attention." Note that each product is different, and you should always read the label before taking any supplements.

Metamucil

Smooth Texture Metamucil is ground into finer particles than Original Texture Metamucil. They both have the same amount of psyllium and the same efficacy. Metamucil can be taken every day as a dietary fiber supplement when used as directed.

One rounded teaspoonful contains: 3.4 grams psyllium fiber, <5 mg sodium, and 9 calories.

Perdiem

Make sure you buy the one that says "no chemicals," because the company also makes a Perdiem with laxative stimulants. I tried the mint flavor, and it wasn't bad at all. You don't mix it with water like you would some of the other products out there. This fiber therapy generally takes effect after 12 hours (but 48 to 72 hours may be required for optimal relief).

Each rounded teaspoonful contains: 4 grams psyllium, 36 mg potassium, 1.8 mg sodium, and 4 calories.

Citrucel (methylcellulose)

"This product does not typically cause bloating," says Walter Coyle, MD, Gastroenterology Program Director with Scripps Clinic. Whereas psyllium and other fibers in food can be broken down by gut bacteria, potentially producing gas and promoting bloating.

Chapter 7

Restaurant Rules

For many people with IBS, including me, eating out can mean intestinal doom. Part of it could be that we tend to eat foods higher in fat when we eat out, part of it could be that we are served larger portions at restaurants, and part of it could be that when we are treating ourselves to a night on the town, we choose foods we normally don't eat. Any or all of these can spell disaster.

We can make ourselves more comfortable during and after eating out by doing a few things.

1. We can make sure we eat only modest amounts (order conservatively, relax, and eat slowly, and remember there are always doggy bags for leftovers).

2. We can choose menu items that aren't too high in fat.

3. We can stick to dishes with which we tend to do well.

Whether or not you eat modest amounts is entirely up to you, but I can help you avoid the rich and greasy items and make menu choices that are lower in fat—no matter where you eat out.

Breakfast at the diner

- Ask the restaurant to make your omelet with egg substitute or one egg blended with a few egg whites.

- Skillet potatoes, made with chunks of potato, should (depending on the restaurant) be a little less greasy than hash browns. You can always request that the potatoes be made with a minimum of oil.

- Enjoy a hot cereal of grits or oatmeal. Grits unfortunately won't contribute any fiber, but oatmeal does.

- A plate of buttermilk pancakes with a strip or two of bacon shouldn't get you into too much trouble, as long as you go light on the butter. If you are choosing between a couple of strips of bacon or two links of breakfast sausage, go for the bacon. Even though we think of bacon as fatty, a typical side order of sausage contains even more fat.

Fast food

For the most part, fast food has a bad reputation—some of it well deserved. But on the up side, some have better options such as grilled chicken sandwiches on whole grain buns, bean burritos, and grilled chicken wraps. You will still be hard-pressed to find a whole serving of fruits or vegetables, or more than a couple of grams fiber, in the typical fast-food offering.

Grilled chicken sandwiches

Most of the fast-food grilled chicken sandwiches I've come across are skinless and pretty tasty. But that's where the uniformity ends. Some come on multigrain buns, some with lettuce and tomato, some dressed in barbecue sauce, and some slathered with creamy honey mustard or even mayonnaise.

- The Grilled Chicken Deluxe at McDonald's has 20 grams fat, 440 calories, and 4 grams fiber. But take away the mayo and the fat grams go down to 5 (and the calories go down to 300).

- The Grilled Chicken Sandwich at Wendy's, which comes with reduced-calorie honey mustard, contains 8 grams fat, 310 calories, and 2 grams fiber.
- The BK Broiler Chicken Sandwich without mayonnaise totals 9 grams fat, 370 calories, and 2 grams fiber.

Fish sandwiches

The good news is that fast-food chains do sell fish. The bad news is that they deep-fry it. But if you eat your fish sandwich without tartar sauce (or at least with most of it scraped off, leaving just enough to wet the bun) you would be surprised to find that when it comes to grams of fat, it can compete with the small hamburger.

- The Burger King fish sandwich (without tartar sauce) contains 14 grams fat, 460 calories, and 3 grams fiber.
- The Filet-O-Fish at McDonald's isn't as big as the Burger King fish sandwich, and without tartar sauce it contains 12 grams fat, 398 calories, and 2 grams fiber.

Baked potatoes

Wendy's offers two baked potato options that are worth biting into. They go a long way toward filling you up and contain at least 8 grams fiber.

- The sour cream and chives potato has 6 grams fat, 380 calories, and 8 grams fiber.
- The broccoli and cheese potato contains 14 grams fat, 470 calories, and 9 grams fiber. Still, fewer than 30 percent of the calories come from fat.

Burgers

When you've just gotta have that burger, be sure it's no larger than a quarter-pounder. And pass up such high-fat toppings and condiments, such as bacon, cheese, and mayonnaise. Try trimmer ones instead, such as mustard, ketchup, barbecue sauce, lettuce, onion, tomato, and hot peppers (all as tolerated). The smallest hamburgers at fast-food chains (the size that comes in the children's meals) are going to be the better bet for a couple of reasons. They have the least amount of beef per square inch of bun. And they are usually made without mayonnaise or other creamy sauces, which is what the bigger, "deluxe" burgers usually come with. Here are two examples:

1. The hamburger at McDonald's has 9 grams fat, 250 calories, 2 grams fiber and 3.5 grams saturated fat; the cheeseburger has 12 grams fat, 300 calories, 2 grams fiber, and 6 grams saturated fat.

2. The Jr. Hamburger at Wendy's has 8 grams fat, 220 calories, 1 gram fiber, and 3 grams saturated fat; the Jr. Cheeseburger totals 11 grams fat, 260 calories, 1 gram fiber, and 5 grams saturated fat.

Entrée Salads

I know, ordering a salad at a fast-food restaurant is almost a sacrilege. But some salads do add some fiber and nutrients while offering a healthful alternative to fried fast food (if you use a light dressing). So if you enjoy salad and if it doesn't provoke IBS symptoms (those with constipation-type IBS may even find that lettuce helps), consider the following:

Chick-fil-A Chargrilled Chicken Garden Salad

180 calories (260 with 2 Tbs. reduced fat raspberry vinaigrette)

6 grams fat (8 grams with raspberry vinaigrette)

3 grams saturated fat

65 mg cholesterol

620 mg sodium (810 mg with raspberry vinaigrette)

3 grams fiber

9 grams carbohydrate (24 grams with raspberry vinaigrette)

22 grams protein

Taco Bell Fresco Style Zesty Chicken Border Bowl (without dressing)

350 calories

8 grams fat

1.5 grams saturated fat

25 mg cholesterol

1,600 mg sodium

10 grams fiber

51 grams carbohydrate

19 grams protein

McDonalds Southwest Salad With Grilled Chicken
(includes cilantro lime glaze and a southwest vegetable/bean blend)

320 calories

9 grams fat

3 grams saturated fat

70 mg cholesterol

970 mg sodium

7 grams fiber

30 grams carbohydrate

30 grams protein

Arby's Martha's Vineyard Salad—not including dressing (includes grilled chicken, diced apples, cherry tomatoes, cheddar, cranberries, and lettuce)

- 277 calories
- 8 grams fat
- 4 grams saturated fat
- 72 mg cholesterol
- 451 mg sodium
- 4 grams fiber
- 24 grams carbohydrate
- 26 grams protein

Carl's Jr. Charbroiled Chicken Salad (with low-fat balsamic dressing)

- 295 calories
- 8.5 grams fat
- 3.5 grams saturated fat
- 75 mg cholesterol
- 1,190 mg sodium
- 5 grams fiber
- 21 grams carbohydrate
- 34 grams protein

Arby's Santa Fe Salad with Grilled Chicken—not including dressing (includes cherry tomatoes, red onion, corn, black beans, cheddar, and lettuce)

- 283 calories
- 9 grams fat
- 4 grams saturated fat
- 72 mg cholesterol
- 521 mg sodium
- 6 grams fiber

21 grams carbohydrate

29 grams protein

McDonalds Asian Salad With Grilled Chicken
(includes mandarin oranges, almonds, edamame, snow peas, and red bell peppers)

300 calories

10 grams fat

1 gram saturated fat

65 mg cholesterol

890 mg sodium

5 grams fiber

23 grams carbohydrate

32 grams protein

Taco Bell and Mexican restaurants

Although the nutritional information that follows is specific to the Taco Bell chain, the food tips may help you in other Mexican fast-food chains or restaurants.

Soft tacos

A soft taco is made with a soft flour tortilla, rather than a crispy (fried) corn tortilla. No matter where you are, a soft taco is usually going to be lower in fat than a crispy taco. At Taco Bell, these are the lower-fat soft tacos:

- Grilled steak soft taco, which has 200 calories, 7 grams total fat, 2.5 grams saturated fat, and 2 grams fiber.
- Grilled chicken soft taco, which has 200 calories, 7 grams total fat, 2.5 grams saturated fat, and 2 grams fiber.

Burritos

Burritos are typically made with large flour tortillas and are not fried (although you can get them fried in some restaurants). Depending on which fillings you choose, they can have double the fat and one-quarter the fiber of the lowest-fat burrito, the bean burrito.

- Bean burrito, which has 370 calories, 12 grams fat, 3.5 grams saturated fat, and 12 grams fiber.
- Grilled chicken burrito, which has 390 calories, 13 grams fat, 4 grams saturated fat, and 3 grams fiber.

Sandwiches

Sandwiches are usually well tolerated (depending on their contents). Request whole wheat bread or rolls to pump up the fiber in your sandwich when you can. If you are bothered by gas and bloating, skip sandwiches stuffed with vegetables.

- Hold the mayo. Order your sandwich with ketchup or mustard. Sometimes Italian delis will lightly wet the bread with an olive oil mixture, which at least adds the more desirable monounsaturated fat. If you must have mayonnaise, ask that they spread it very lightly.
- Choose leaner meats. Roast chicken, roast turkey, and roast beef are all great choices; a lean ham will also do well.
- When it comes to chicken, shrimp, or tuna salad, you are better off enjoying a light version made at home. Restaurants and delis usually make these salads with generous amounts of mayonnaise.

Pizza

I have to admit that I'm partial to pizza. My family probably orders or makes pizza once a week. Nearly everybody has a favorite pizza chain, some of which make greasier pizza than others. Basically, the more authentically Italian your pizza is (made with a breadier crust and light on the cheese), the lower in fat the crust will be. That's half the battle. The other half is how you top that crust. Don't use gobs of cheese, and avoid fatty, spicy meats, which can get you into trouble very quickly. If at all possible, order your pizza with vegetable toppings you like and tolerate well. If you are a meat lover, your best bet is Canadian bacon or lean ham.

Another important trick to pizza is quitting while you're ahead. It's easy to eat slice after slice of pizza until you are stuffed. Stick to two large slices in one sitting. If you are still hungry, have some fruit, a bowl of soup, or a green salad as tolerated.

The rotisserie restaurant

- Enjoy sliced turkey breast or lean ham with new potatoes, steamed vegetables, and hot cinnamon apples and your bill will ring up to around 595 calories, with 9 grams fat and 2 grams saturated fat.

- If you opt for the roasted chicken, skip the skin (that's where most of the fat is) or just eat a few bites of the crispy bits you can't resist and toss the rest.

- Pass up such creamy side dishes as creamed spinach and ask for the baked new potatoes or sweet potatoes, zucchini marinara, rice pilaf, red beans and rice, steamed vegetables, or fresh fruit.

- The meat loaf sandwich (without cheese) should keep your fat in check, especially if you have it with a low-fat soup and/or fruits and vegetables.

- Chicken noodle soup (and most other clear soups) with corn bread can make a nice light lunch or dinner.

The steakhouse

The trouble with eating at steakhouses is that many foods are deep fried and/or high in fat, and most of the time you saddle up to cowboy-sized servings. You can plan ahead and make yourself more comfortable after the meal by finding items you enjoy that are better, leaner choices, and making sure you eat only until you are comfortably full. Don't overdo it.

- The lean cuts of beef available at steakhouses are usually sirloin or filet mignon (the fatter cuts are rib eye, prime rib, porterhouse, and T-bone).

- Order the "petite" or "junior" portions of meat when available.

- Trim all visible fat from whichever cut of meat you choose.

- Have your meat dish with lots of vegetables that you tolerate well (beans if you are able). The vegetables will help fill you up so you won't be tempted to overdo the meat, and the vegetables and beans help boost fiber totals.

- Eat side dishes that you tolerate well and that are lower in fat to help balance out the beef. These might include a clear broth or tomato-based soup, baked potato (modest on butter and sour cream) or mashed potatoes, broccoli, beans, rice pilaf, dinner roll, corn bread, and cinnamon apples.

Contemporary cuisine tips

- Grilled or roasted chicken and fish are two of the healthiest things you can order at many restaurants.

- Ask that the skin be removed from your chicken before it is prepared.

- Order leaner cuts of beef. Top sirloin and filet mignon are good choices.

- High-fat, buttery, or creamy sauces should be garnishes, not large portions of the meal. Ask for half as much of these sauces when ordering pasta or meat dishes.

- If you really want a dish that is sauteed or simmered in cream or butter, ask that it be simmered in wine or broth instead.

- Ask to substitute marinara, marsala, or wine sauces for cream and butter sauces that come with chicken, fish, or pasta.

Casual cuisine tips

- Ask for salad dressing on the side. This way, you decide how much to add to your salad.

- Ask for grilled chicken instead of fried.

- Some of our favorite comfort foods, such as pot roast or turkey dinners, are actually some of the lower-fat and better tolerated entrees at restaurants.

- Grilled chicken breast is always a good choice at a restaurant.

- Grilled fish is a great dinner choice. Not only does fish contain beneficial omega-3 fatty acids, it is also the type of dinner we tend to not make for ourselves at home.

Chinese restaurants

In general, you may have to avoid items marked hot and spicy. Garlic, curry, hot peppers, and ginger can give some people problems. You can easily avoid the hot peppers and curry by ordering items that don't contain them, but it is more difficult to avoid garlic and ginger, both of which seem to be in almost everything. If you can tolerate a little of either, then perhaps all you need to do is avoid the dishes that have ginger or garlic in their titles (such as garlic shrimp or ginger beef).

The other group of menu items to steer clear of is deep-fried items. Similar to most rich foods, they can wreak havoc on your intestines. Stir-fried dishes tend to be well tolerated by most with IBS, but I would guess that the higher the amount of oil used in the stir-fry, the greater the potential discomfort and aftereffects.

Japanese restaurants

IBS sufferers usually do well with rice, fish, and grilled or broiled meats, so all those wonderful grilled dishes in Japanese restaurants are probably a good bet. Japanese noodle soups and the standard miso soup should also be fine.

Tempura, the one dish that causes me trouble in Japanese restaurants, is also my favorite (funny how that works). But I've learned that if I only eat four pieces or so (about half an order), I seem to be fine. Of course, I'm eating the tempura with soup and lots of rice. If I eat the entire entrée (which is easy to do because it tastes so wonderful), I'm done for.

Italian restaurants

If you are not bothered by tomatoes, you will have many choices at Italian restaurants. Any entrée made with lean meat or vegetables and marinara sauce might work well. If you like pasta with cream sauce, keep your portions very small and enjoy less rich (and higher fiber if possible) side dishes with it, such as bread, soup, and vegetables.

Mediterranean restaurants

People in the Mediterranean like their fish and shellfish. Fish is usually well tolerated by people with IBS, and it's even better for you if you eat it with some rice and in-season vegetables. Olive oil and olives are also a big part of Mediterranean cuisine. This might only be a problem if you eat a large amount of olive oil at one time.

I love going to restaurants. What's not to like? But when you have IBS, you can pay dearly for the fun of eating out. If you follow the tips in this chapter, you may well spare yourself future discomfort.

Index

About the Author

Elaine Magee is positively passionate about changing the way America eats, one recipe at a time! Through her national column, The Recipe Doctor (appearing in newspapers such as the *Bay Area News Group, Hartfort Courant, Democrat and Chronicle, The News-Gazette, The Lancaster New Era, The Honolulu Advertiser,* and others), Elaine has been performing recipe "makeovers" for a decade now. Elaine is the author of more than 25 books on nutrition and healthy cooking, including her most recent, *Food Synergy.* Elaine's medical nutrition series including *Tell Me What to Eat If I Have Diabetes, Tell Me What to Eat If I Have Acid Reflux,* and *Tell Me What to Eat If I Have Headaches and Migraines* (and others)—has sold hundreds of thousands of copies and are now being distributed all over the world, including China, Russia, Spain, Indonesia, and Arabic countries.

Elaine is a nutrition expert/writer for *Webmd.com* and magazines across the country and appears frequently on radio, educational videos, and television shows. She has appeared on *View From the Bay, Good Morning Texas,* the *Fine Living Network,* and the CBS Evening News. Elaine graduated as the Nutrition Science Department's "Student of the Year" from San Jose State University with a BS in nutrition with a minor in chemistry. She also obtained her master's degree in public health nutrition from UC Berkeley and is a registered dietitian.

Contributor:

Christine Frissora, MD, is an associate professor of medicine and gastroenterologist at the NY-Cornell Medical Center and specializes in functional disorders of the GI tract. Dr. Frissora has lectured across the nation to doctors, nurses, and other health professionals. She is widely published, with a national reputation for treating IBS and related disorders.